HOW TO HEAL YOUR BFRB

HOW TO HEAL YOUR BFRB

*4 Steps to Stop Compulsive
Skin Picking, Hair Pulling & More*

Lauren Inés Ruiz Bloise

Bloise Books

Copyright © 2023 Lauren Inés Ruiz Bloise

Published in the United States. All rights reserved. No part of this publication may be reproduced or transmitted in any form without written permission from the publisher/author. It is illegal to copy this book, post it to a website, or distribute it by any means. This content is registered with the US Copyright Office. Legal action may be sought against persons selling unauthorized files/portions of this book.

To notify of illegal distribution, please email: contact@healyourBFRB.com.

Paperback ISBN: 978-1-7364617-1-6
Hardcover ISBN: 978-1-7364617-2-3
eISBN: 978-1-7364617-0-9

Design and cover by the author

Typefaces include Arno Pro, Myriad Pro, Adobe Handwriting Ernie, Bubblegum Baby, Plants, and Dotuku Dingbats.

Second edition

Although every effort was made to ensure the information presented here was correct at time of publication, the publisher/author does not assume and hereby disclaims any liability for any loss, damage, or disruption caused by errors or omissions, whether such errors or omissions result from negligence, accident, or any other cause.

This book is not intended as a substitute for the medical advice of physicians. The reader should regularly consult a physician in matters relating to their health and particularly with respect to any symptoms that may require diagnosis or medical attention.

No affiliation exists with any of the sites, brands, or apps mentioned (other than healyourBFRB.com).

The publisher/author has no responsibility for the persistence of the URLs in this publication and does not guarantee the websites will remain accurate or appropriate over time.

Contents

Pre-Steps

Why Determination Alone Will Not Heal Your BFRB   5
My BFRB Story   6
Challenging the Mania Mind   9
Why We Pick   20
Why Do You Want to Stop?   21
Recognize What You're Actually Doing   23
Your Basics   24
Other Diagnoses   24
Treatments Are Effective   25

The Steps

Step 1: Increase Your Awareness via a Log   29
Step 2: Identify Triggers and Keep a Thorough List   51
Step 3: Establish Protectors and Keep a Thorough List   65
Step 4: Practice Protectors   201

Post Steps

Track Your Improvement   227
How Long Does This Take?   230
What Healing Means   232
Relapse   233
When to Stop Following These Steps   234
More Logging and Listing Options   235

End

Endnotes   239
Selected Bibliography   243
Resources   243
Acknowledgements   245
About the Author   245
Contact   245
More BFRB Guide   245
Review & Recommend   247

Before Starting

As you likely know, BFRB stands for "body-focused repetitive behavior." It's an umbrella term for disorders that include dermatillomania (skin picking), trichotillomania (hair pulling), onychophagy (nail biting), and dermatophagia (skin biting).

To Heal Yours with This Guide . . .

Don't stop reading just because you start feeling good. Hope and anticipation of relief can be confused with healing, except these will only keep you from picking for a little while.

Don't stop reading because you think you get it. Even if you start to predict what's next, or already know about some of the topics discussed, the nuances can make the difference between healing and continuing to struggle.

Have a note app or physical notebook ready. If your default app isn't great, I highly recommend Nction.so or Google Keep. They're free, and notes can be accessed via a computer, tablet, or phone, so they're flexible. If you prefer pen and paper, find a notebook, possibly one that fits in a purse or large pocket.

Get a note app or notebook ready now, or as soon as you can.

Replace "pick" with "pull" or "chew" as needed. Ideally, I would tailor this guide to every BFRB, but that would be a much longer book. Picking is referred to most often, but regardless of your BFRB, this guide is for you too.

If You're Not a Reader, to Help You Finish the BFRB Guide . . .

Read just a tiny bit daily (or most days), like one page. If you have resistance to that, read half, or read *one paragraph*. This maintains forward momentum.

Try your daily reading in the morning, afternoon, or night till you find a time you can stick to.

Bookmark/highlight the exact line or word you leave off at so you don't lose your enthusiasm re-reading to find your spot.

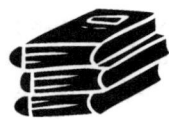

Pre-Steps

Why Determination Alone Will Not Heal Your BFRB

My BFRB Story

Challenging the Mania Mind

Why We Pick

Why Do You Want to Stop?

Recognize What You're Actually Doing

Your Basics

Other Diagnoses

Treatments Are Effective

Why Determination Alone Will Not Heal Your BFRB

Simply determining to *not pick* is one of our few tools against dermatillomania for months, years, or decades. It goes like this: "I will not pick ever again—starting now." We exercise this determination with our willpower (aka, self-control).

But willpower is not enough.

You've tried it. I've tried it.

Willpower can be compared to a muscle. After a lot of exercise, it must rest, or it'll give out on you. You can also think of it as being like a well. As you use it, the water dips lower, and the well gets emptier.

After determining to not pick, you may be able to use willpower to keep yourself from picking for a while, but each time you tap into your willpower, you have less of it, till you reach the bottom of the well so to speak, and you eventually pick as badly as ever.

Not that I want to give you a limited view of your self-control. Research explains that self-control is affected by our beliefs on it[1] (i.e., believing you have it in vast supply versus that you're a person with low self-control makes a difference).

Self-control is also affected by how we frame things (e.g., seeing something as easy or hard to do affects how easy or hard it is). And, just like a well refills when it rains, your willpower reserves replenish through rest, nutritious food, relaxation, and more.

However, when it comes to BFRBs, trying to stop with sheer force of will alone *has* failed.

It is not the path of least resistance.

You *must* call up willpower against your dermatillomania, but willpower is only a small aid that comes into play once you have more advanced tools, like the ones described in this guide.

My BFRB Story: Dermatillomania

You might read this to see how similar or different our stories are, for camaraderie, and to learn a little more about BFRBs—or, feel free to skip it.

The Start

In early middle school, I began leaning over the bathroom sink to get as freakishly close to the mirror as I could and pop the pimples I now had (thanks to puberty). I would do this for so long that my mom would come check whether I was OK. She would ask me to stop; I wouldn't budge. "You're marking up your face!" she'd yell, losing her patience after trying to pull me away so often.

I ignored her for months, until I started seeing signs that she was right.

But then, when I tried to stop, I couldn't.

◆

Though I targeted many things, blemishes and ingrown hairs were my main focus, no matter how tiny or nearly non-existent. My face was my main area of concern. An "attack" there would bring me the most anguish. But other places were perpetually picked at too, including my legs, armpits, chest, pubic area, back, breasts, shoulders, arms, and neck.

Others target their fingers or lips, feet or cheeks, eczema or psoriasis, bug bites, large scabs, or perceived imperfections. There seem to be as many variations of this thing as there are names for it—*dermatillomania, excoriated acne, compulsive skin picking (CSP), skin picking disorder (SPD), obsessive skin picking, neurotic excoriation* . . .

All body-focused repetitive behaviors, e.g., hair pulling, nail biting, skin biting, nose picking (rhinotillexomania), share characteristics but have specifics all their own, and it's also individual from person to person. Personally, I don't feel tingling before an urge, and I don't sniff or eat anything like some do, although there's absolutely no judgment here—about anything.

Over Time

At night, I'd stay awake with a flashlight to my legs in my darkened room till my eyes ached after picking for who knows how long. I'd simply walk by a mirror and become trapped.

Once out of high school, I'd be sitting at my desk in the middle of work and get up, as if possessed, to find a mirror.

I would fight with myself: *Walk away... please stop!* Negotiate: *Once I get that one... I'll never pick again!*

I'd scatter sewing pins, bobby pins, tweezers, and more across my bathroom floor, dropping them to get a better angle, before I would snatch them up to poke more, leaving myself red and raw. I'd cry and feel despair, incompetence, and anger in the face of my excoriation.

Every now and then, I would be able to pop only a few things and walk away, simply reminding myself I didn't want to do this. My dermatillomania would fade into the background. The whole thing wouldn't be such a problem.

Then it'd return to the forefront, full force, becoming one of the main issues in my life again. *Why can't I stop?!*

I tried so many ways and so many times to stop. Usually I would just determine to never do it again, but sometimes I got creative. For example, when I was twenty-five, I paid my partner at the time money whenever I picked: $5 for my face and $1 for elsewhere. I shelled out around $150 and owed much more before I gave up on that idea.

Turning Point

Whereas before I'd be surprised at how well most wounds healed up, in my mid to late twenties, as my skin's collagen production began slowing (as it does around this age), every bad session left a permanent mark. I began losing the hope I had somehow maintained for nearly two decades.

I actually am *stuck with this. I'm going to helplessly watch my skin deteriorate over the years.*

But I hadn't given in yet. I made a list of therapists after searching online. How had I not sought one out before?

Most of the therapists were far away. Few specialized in BFRBs. All were too expensive. *Oh yeah.*

Stuck in the cycle as I was, I would look it up every few years, see it was out of my reach, and forget about it. But if not now, when? I'd make myself be able to afford it.

Finally, I found a therapist who offered a payment plan and a therapy that was effective for at least some BFRBers. I called to make an appointment, but...

We couldn't get our schedules to line up.

Time passed, and then, when I called again... the therapist told me she was booked.

I remembered what I had heard others say: "You can heal yourself" (a general, non-BFRB statement); you don't need anyone else. Well, I certainly did, because I *hadn't* been able to figure it out. This woman was my last hope. If I couldn't get an appointment with her, I was sure I would keep picking.

Nothing had worked.

If I could figure this out on my own, though, I could save a lot of money. With my newfound resolve, I kept working on a few things related to my dermatillomania without thinking much about it.

One night, when I realized I had been doing damn well, I added up my picking, which I'd now been keeping track of. For most of my life, I picked daily. One full day without picking was a success. A few days was a feat. And more than that was impossible. In a matter of months, my picking had dropped by a third, and it was still improving.

How?!

I thought about what I had been doing. I broke it down into a few steps. My next thought was *I know how to do this!*

◆

I dealt with the worst of my dermatillomania for about seventeen years before these steps.

Some have decades of picking or pulling on me, and others have only been doing it for a few months; some have it much worse, and others are affected a little less. Regardless, the following steps apply.

What's your BFRB story? Do you deal with just one BFRB, or a few? When did it start for you?

Challenging the Mania Mind: Should You Stop?

Before we get to the steps, it'll help if we're on the same page.

Some of us are on board with stopping 100%. Even though we feel we can't, we *want* to stop altogether. (I recognize that while we don't want to pick . . . we want to pick—let's put that aside here.) Personally, I desperately wanted to stop, but I wasn't sure I *should*, at least not completely.

Though I'll mostly focus on blemishes in this section, whether you're a picker, puller, or biter, please read on; you can apply the following to whatever you do. And at times I'll address BFRBs other than blemish-focused dermatillomania directly.

Experts Are Conflicted

During my dermatillomania-fueled research into skin care, I learned that it's OK to extract certain blemishes.

I read articles and watched videos on how to do it properly. While there are different methods, it usually involves tools, correct finger positioning, proper pressure, pulling and then pushing of the skin, sterilization, steaming, and more—the point is to minimize adverse effects.

If you've done the same research I have, you may *also* have learned that you should **never extract pimples yourself.**

Interesting.

I wanted to stop altogether, but I was worried some things would never go away without my help. I'd miraculously let a few things be for some time, and they were lingering.

And here were professionals saying I could and maybe *should* pick (or, technically, "extract"). So for many years, I ignored the experts who strongly advised against it, and I would fall back on picking the "right" way.

Finally I learned which is true.

For the optimal health and beauty of the skin, one should *never* pick . . .

Especially with dermatillomania present.

Why Skin Pickers, Especially, Shouldn't Pick

At some point, I wrote a thorough plan on how, what, and when to pick so I could do it "right." I called it "My New Skin Plan: Picking Is OK." A psychological breakthrough (*because I'm a genius*)—if I gave myself permission to pick, it would alleviate the pressure I put on myself and keep me from doing it as much.

So I learned about the different types of blemishes and how spots can be roughly categorized as A's, B's, and C's, the idea being that A's can be extracted as part of grooming, while B's are best helped along via skin care products (or ignored) but should not be extracted. C is normal, clear skin.

For example:

A—A big pustule that has fully come to a head (many erroneously call pustules "whiteheads"); a big shallow blackhead.

B—A pustule of any size that's not at a head; a medium or small blackhead (aka an "open comedone"); any closed comedone (a true "whitehead," it looks like a white bump under the skin); skin-colored bumps; shaving bumps; most ingrown hairs; scabs; cysts.

C—Clear skin.

My goal was to view my skin like a "normal" person. If I got a zit, I would assess whether I should pop it, and if it wasn't ready, I'd leave it alone. I'd let the tiny things be, regardless of how long they wanted to stick around. I'd display spots with or without some makeup, not caring they were there. I'd focus on my clothing style and posture—on the person I am and the things I wanted to accomplish and experience.

This was my vision.

I didn't follow my New Skin Plan for a single day.

The dermatillo-*mania* mind (or trichotillo-*mania* mind), as I call it, has a way of skewing our thinking, so I couldn't distinguish between what I could "safely" pick and what I should leave alone.

Psychologists have various terms for the factors that play in, but for our purposes, simplifying it to "mania mind" works.

I would see the tiniest head and call a spot ready.

I'd sense something beneath the surface and go for it.

And when picking "right" didn't extract it, I didn't leave it be like *all* experts advise. I'd try whatever I could to get it out, whatever tools, whatever pressure, clean hands and skin or not, the future integrity of my skin be damned.

Or I'd successfully pick that one thing, but rather than back away and call it a win, I'd hunt for anything else I could find, ready or not.

The plan I wrote could work for someone without skin picking disorder, who gets rid of pimples as part of normal grooming.

But if we, as pickers, have the mentality that we can pick *some* things, the impulse to pick *everything*, any way possible, is too easy to fall into.

So my recommendation is this:

Never, ever, pick.

You can't say right now you'll never pick again, I understand that—we haven't even gotten to the steps—I'm saying *decide* that to **never** do it is your aim.

I really like this comparison:

Some argue that drinking has health benefits, but whether a certain amount of wine or beer a day is healthy or not is irrelevant for an alcoholic, because the alcoholic's excess obliterates *any* benefits. For a true alcoholic, the recommended solution is to quit altogether. A true alcoholic can never be a social drinker.

Similarly, proper extraction is irrelevant for us—whether some experts recommend it, whether we know people who do it, or whether *sometimes* it turns out OK for us.

Some non-BFRBers have a zero-picking mentality anyway, so it's not unheard of, and again, it is what many experts advise.[2]

Thankfully, the alcoholic doesn't need to drink to find health, just as we don't need to pick to have nice skin. Quite the opposite.

◆

On that note—if you don't want to wait around for a certain spot to go away on its own, or if you think it won't, having a dermatologist or esthetician perform an extraction is ideal.

Those with certain types of acne or skin conditions might look into routine extractions. Not all professionals are equal, so read reviews and call to ask questions.

While you may assume extractions are not accessible to you (maybe because of the cost), you may find they actually are accessible if you look into them.

♦

Making routine appointments with a professional is advisable for other types of BFRBers too, for example, someone with trich can make brow-waxing appointments.

But avoiding all grooming related to BFRBs may be impractical.

If you're someone with trich, and you have an obvious stray hair on your chin or brow, it may be unrealistic to book an appointment for that. If you pick at your fingers, it may be impractical to book a manicure every time the skin around your nails frays.

Whatever your reason for grooming yourself, if you have, let's say, trichotillomania or some combination of BFRBs, let these questions guide you:

- **Is this something a non-BFRBer would target?**

  A non-BFRBer might pluck between their brows, but they would almost never pluck any hair from their head, lashes, or the brows themselves.

- **How would a non-BFRBer groom this?**

  An obvious piece of frayed skin around the fingers would likely get snipped with nail clippers.

- **How should *I* groom this?**

  While those with healthier grooming behaviors are a guide for what you might do, you must accommodate for the fact that you do have a BFRB.

If you try your hand at normal grooming, you might as well still view most targets through the lens of "never pick," "never pull," or "never chew," that's how narrow *any* exceptions will be.

And, perhaps you ultimately do decide to *never* groom anything related to your particular BFRB on your own.

◆

When you decide to never go for it, there's no more dangerous or uncomfortable back and forth. *Should I get that? Can I get that?*

No more deliberating.

The *mania* mind has much less leverage—because now you know the answer: *No, I shouldn't get that.*

Anyway, no matter what you decide, it's pointless.

Why It's Pointless Anyway

When I saw something pickable, it needed to be obliterated, removed, dug out. But the incentive started fading when I learned the following.

1

When a pimple is picked, the contents can spread over the skin's surface and enter neighboring pores, causing **more pimples**. This is true even if it's a tiny scrape, scratch, or pop, or a small blemish.

> *The body intends for this stuff to be contained as it works on taking care of the issue (by absorbing the gunk or letting it dry up). When we open a pimple, we ignore that mechanism.*

Suppose you sanitize your hands, tools, and skin, before and immediately after, and minimize this somewhat—there are still a few problems, ones that are out of our control:

2

Technically, the pore we see on the skin is the opening to the *follicular canal*, which is beneath the surface. With pressure, the sides of the follicular canal holding a blemish can rupture. When the canal ruptures, its contents spread into neighboring canals beneath the surface, again causing **more pimples**.

3

An extraction can often be incomplete,[3] leaving behind some of the contents (dead skin, infection, sebum, bacteria), so even if the spot looks better for a bit, it **redevelops** soon enough.

4

By applying pressure, we may be pushing contents deeper *down* into the canal (despite our effort to do the opposite), so the blemish again **redevelops**, often bigger and angrier, now that it's been irritated.

We've all picked at something unnoticeable only to make it obvious—this is why.

5

These aren't the only reasons spots come back. For example, the wall, or sac, of a sebaceous cyst may require surgical removal to keep it from filling back up.[4] Good luck trying to squeeze one of these cysts and get it to go away (*please* don't attempt to get the wall out yourself—it can be dangerous).

◆

If no matter how hard I tried, I wasn't getting *all* of the stuff out, and I was creating more pimples, by spreading the contents above and beneath the surface—whether it was the same spot, or a new one, a wound or a scar, I would have something on me.

Even if I picked.

This all led to an epiphany:

> Picking does not achieve what I want anyway.

I also realized whether it was when I was on my period, or the next time I got stressed, ate the wrong thing, got sweaty, or washed my skin improperly, *pimples came back*. Ingrown hairs and shaving bumps, too, reappeared.

For years I'd attempt to pick at everything till I had no spots. Once I had a clean slate, my problem would be solved.

Success, right?

No.

A "clean slate" is impossible, yet over and over my *mania* mind encouraged me to forget that I had yet to achieve one.

Similarly, pulling an irregular hair won't keep others from appearing. Cuticles will become frayed again. Lip biting/picking, like blemish picking, exacerbates the endless cycle by giving you more things to target.

> Part of healing is accepting you'll have pickable, pullable, or chewable things on your body, from time to time and probably always to some extent.

For me, the realization that it's inevitable—and normal—to have pickable things on me helped shift my perfectionist mentality, which had led to self-criticism and wasn't helping me heal.

> *Don't be fooled into thinking some have flawless skin. You might have seen a few people who seem to, but even they get spots here and there. While I watched* TV, *I'd notice how certain lighting emphasized acne scars or blemishes on an actress—someone society deemed the epitome of beauty, or more importantly, who even I was taken with.*
>
> *I thought back on the crushes I'd had on people with acne and scarring. The relationships. And how these things never deterred me.*
>
> *Even if someone out there has zero pickable things, the majority of us just do, and flawless skin is not a necessary ingredient for beauty or love, which by the way, is so much more complex than just what we look like.*

That said, there's another reason BFRBers should never pick. Avoiding life-threatening infections that start out by picking a seemingly harmless spot is a *tremendous* reason, but that's not even the one I have in mind.

Why Professional Appointments May Just Be Worth It

Since at-home extractions, especially done by a skin picker, can so easily go wrong, aside from being pointless, they can also lead to:

- Enlarged pores
- Volume loss
- Discoloration
- Scars (rolling, boxcar, icepick, and/or hypertrophic)

> *Even if left alone, a blemish might scar or discolor, but with improper extractions, it's more likely to happen and to be worse.*[5]

The issues that result from skin picking disorder can be helped with procedures, such as fillers, laser treatments, dermabrasion, microdermabrasion, and peels.

But not only are these treatments expensive and intensive, some of the consequences are hard to reverse with current technologies even if you have a high budget. Additionally, the enlarged pores and scarring mentioned above become more obvious with age, as enlarged pores begin to distend, and collagen and elastin continue to taper off.

> The most effective, and affordable, way to have "nice" skin isn't a cosmetic procedure that *restores* it; it's to *keep* it as nice as we can.

For these reasons, performing extractions yourself at home to save money is not worth it. Any money you save will be funneled into reparative treatments (if you're intent on trying to restore your skin), which may not even be as successful as you'd like.

I do encourage you to look into these procedures if you think they might make you happier. However, in all cases, these will only be sensible to invest in once your BFRB is radically reduced.

For hair pullers, chronic pulling can lead to "shocking" the hair follicle into slow regrowth and in some cases to permanent hair loss.[6] For hair, laser treatments or a hair transplant is an option (thankfully, in many cases, patience and hair care are too).

As I said earlier, there's so much more to beauty, to love—to life—than what we look like! But there's nothing wrong with wanting to look our personal best.

It's discouraging when we pick, pull, or bite so badly that we're sure we've added scarring or disrupted collagen, but the good news is that any session we prevent by beginning to heal our BFRB will stop additional consequences.

What Happens When You Leave Your Skin Alone

When I began reducing my picking, I had more pimples than ever. Because pimples can take weeks to form,[7] as you stop picking regularly, you too may see pimples add up as everything you've pushed down and around is let to run its course.

But once my face cleared, my skin looked *better than ever*.

If you've never stopped picking long enough to see a blemish resolve on its own (or if it's been so long that you've forgotten), here's what you can look forward to.

A **pustule** begins to scab and get smaller and flatter until it's a dried granule. The granule falls away on its own or is exfoliated through gentle, routine skin care. Discoloration will fade on its own or can be helped along. Cystic acne will heal about the same.

It's beautiful.

A **closed comedone** (a true "whitehead") and things like it can be diminished over time with skin care products, if they don't dry up like described above.

When it comes to **sebaceous filaments** (those things on the nose and elsewhere), your best bet is to keep the pores tight by using products, rather than by picking, since in the case of sebaceous filaments, they'll absolutely return.

Blackheads can be reduced and *prevented* with products as well.

◆

So, with the *right* care and products (specifics will be given later), not only can we help resolve existing conditions faster and better, we can also *help prevent them* (not just breakouts but frayed cuticles, peeling nails, and more).

Here's a mantra for you: treat, don't pick.

While professional extractions are an option, and some spots could use them, more often than not, blemishes resolve on their own. Yes, some can take weeks to months to disappear, but many go away in just a day or two, if we let them.

And remember, pimples, bumps, frays, different textures, these things are normal and OK, and impossible to avoid. Start making peace with this fact now.

Heal Not Only Your BFRB, but Your Skin Too

While preventing blemishes forevermore is unrealistic, if you have severe acne, or even mild or moderate breakouts, alongside healing your dermatillomania, start or keep working on identifying the **underlying cause**.

Most likely, your severe acne is a symptom, a cry for attention from some part of your system, while mild to moderate breakouts are, if not signaling a pressing issue, an attempt to regulate or detoxify something that's out of whack or not ideal for your body.

That said, when it comes to breakouts, you hear such different advice because *many* factors *can* cause or contribute to acne. So the factors causing yours may not be causing someone else's.

I list a few of my favorite acne resources at the end of this guide and touch upon blemishes in a few different areas throughout.

◆

Perhaps for you it's dry skin, psoriasis, eczema, or some other skin condition that exacerbates your picking—please start or keep working on identifying what it is and what helps manage it. Make this a priority.

Convinced, Or . . . ?

If you aren't convinced on a zero-picking goal, acknowledge your worries. Maybe you're afraid things *won't* go away on their own and you're hesitant about the idea of booking professional extractions—accept that this is where you are. In the meantime, observe your skin as well as your behavior around "grooming-related," "normal" picking (or other BFRB grooming).

How often does it go away faster? How often does it just get worse?

How often are you able to groom only the one or few things you think are appropriate and then stop once you're done, or halt if you realize you're not helping the situation?

How often does the thought of going to see if anything is "ready" have you picking anything and everything unrestrained?

◆

In the end, you may decide to continue extracting *some* blemishes. Maybe this works for you. It never did for me, though. The same goes for other skin pickers who were able to heal their BFRB only when they came to terms with the fact that *picking is pointless*.

We realize soon enough that it's harmful, but the breakthrough is that it's **pointless**.

If you're undecided or unconvinced, you're welcome to start the steps anyway—in fact, please do.

If we're on the same page, *great*—please get rid of any tools, e.g., the comedone extractor and the magnification mirror (which, by the way, distorts the reality of your skin). And I do mean get rid of them right now. Any money you spent on them isn't worth the adverse effects you've caused, and will cause, with these items.

> "Don't go for the one, for the one, for the one."
> —Gaelic Storm (about drinking)

> "Once you pop, you can't stop."
> —Original Pringles' slogan (about Pringles... but it might as well be about dermatillomania)

Why We Pick

The desire to *get it out* or have it *gone* may seem like the main factor behind this compulsion, but usually, the bigger force is this:

The desire to **escape**.

No matter how subtle—but especially as it builds—any unease, stress, anxiety, boredom, worry, tiredness, or *insert unpleasant emotion* that we feel leads us to escape via the easiest means: BFRBs and other destructive behaviors, which offer us stimulation, relaxation, or distraction, and make us feel better—if for the time being.

Another way to put it is that we pick to regulate how we're feeling.

We generally engage in BFRBs because we're trying **to help ourselves to feel better**. From this viewpoint, hopefully you can see that BFRB part of yourself with compassion.

But there are ways to deal that don't have mental or physical repercussions (these better ways will be discussed later).

By escaping into our BFRB so often, our BFRB has become habitual. (I'd never say a BFRB is "just a bad habit," but habit is an important component of it, as I'll explain later.) So, on the one hand, we pick to escape, and on the other, we pick out of hardwired habit.

◆

Another way to answer "why do we engage in BFRBs?" is that it's likely a mix of our biology, psychology, and experience.[8] The details of that won't be covered in this guide, since you can heal without knowing them, but sources and resources are listed at the end if you're curious.

Why Do You Want to Stop?

A strong why is one of the most powerful motivators we have toward change. Reasons BFRBers state for wanting to stop include: being able to confidently wear tank tops and shorts, rather than hiding with long sleeves and pants; being able to wear any hairstyle, rather than being limited to styles that cover marks or bald spots; not needing to wear makeup when they don't feel like it; to look their best for a special event, such as a wedding or party; or to have more time.

These reasons count.

But in the moment of an urge, picking often entices us more than whether we can wear certain clothes or hairstyles or looking our best for an event. That means our reason for stopping must be *bigger* than our desire to pick.

To find this bigger reason, we have to go beyond appearances and anything surface level, and dive into our deepest desires and values.

Below are examples of whys that may win against the momentary satisfaction of picking, pulling, or chewing. Maybe you want to stop because:

- You'll be **setting a good example** for some young person, perhaps your child, so they can be an overall happier kid and adult.

    The idea is that you care more about the quality of life of this person, who may model your behavior, than about eradicating a pimple or hair.

- You'll have **more time** to dedicate to building a new business, so you can leave your current job and live a **freer, more peaceful life**.

    Having sufficient time to create a happier life is more compelling than just "having more time."

- You'll feel more confident dating and showing your true physical self to potential partners, which will set you up better for **finding love**, again or for the first time.

Acceptance, connection, and companionship are deeper drivers.

- You'll feel confident putting yourself out there so you can make more friends or connections, or do meaningful things in the world, which will make you **more fulfilled**.

Not being held back by your appearance is more important than the actual improvement of your appearance.

- You'll **be in control**. This will raise your self-esteem and make you feel more like the you, you want to be, or already are at your best.

You, your self-concept, and doing right by yourself matters more than giving in to your dermatillomania or trichotillomania.

◆

We all have different desires and values, so you have to find what resonates with you. I recommend you record what you hope to gain from healing your BFRB, right now (be it in a list or a rambling journal entry). You don't have to, but it'll only help.

As you write, enjoy it, feel it.

And dig for a why till you find one that hits home.

A last note is that your reason may evolve. Let's say that young person in your life does not develop a BFRB, so you no longer have to be their role model in that sense, or you find a partner who just doesn't care about the state of your skin, hair, or nails. That's wonderful! But it may mean it's time to unearth another why.

◆

Your reasons for stopping will be your North Star throughout your healing anytime you feel lost or unmotivated.

So, beyond the obvious reasons, why *do* you want to stop? What will it mean for you and your life?

Recognize What You're Actually Doing

Some are already keenly aware of the scars, marks, and patches, but some aren't—at least, perhaps, not entirely.

As BFRBers, we become so used to zooming in on one zone in the fit of picking or pulling that we miss the big picture. We might deem a tiny spot as meaningful, and obvious wounds or patches as not that bad, as we gloss over them to pick or pull more.

But when we step *back*, rather than lean in viciously close, we get a more balanced view.

Before starting, I recommend you take in your target areas to help you see what you're *actually* doing. Refocus your eyes so you're looking at an entire area at once. Do it part by part: your face, your chest, your arms, and so on.

For some of you, this may mean standing in front of a large mirror while holding a hand-held mirror to the back of your head, or stretching your arms out and taking a good look at your nails and fingers—your hands—as a whole.

To further help you recognize what you're actually doing, snap pictures of the tools or tissue paper you throw about after a session, or of a pile of hair you've pulled.

◆

When you shift your perspective and see the whole of your beauty and your behavior, good and bad things happen. Both the good and bad feelings are aids for the growth and healing you want.

That said, these scars, marks, and patches do *not* make up the whole of who you are, and they will get better with time (you can also do things, like the procedures discussed earlier and more, to improve them once your BFRB is under control).

Your Basics

I couldn't write a guide on how to stop body-focused repetitive behaviors and *not* discuss the basics. The basics are part of your foundation as a person, and the correlation between your foundation and how much you pick, pull, or bite isn't small. It's not even medium-sized.

It's gigantic.

When I say the "basics," I'm talking about how well you **eat** and **sleep** and how often you **move** your body. These basics help counteract not only disease and signs of aging, but also stress, anxiety, depression, and, well, body-focused repetitive behaviors.

So take inventory as you begin reading the steps:

What do you eat and when? How do you feel after? What about if you eat too little? Too much?

Do you feel unmotivated, irritable, low? *Do urges increase?*

How much do you sleep and when? Do you usually get enough sleep? Or rarely? How do you feel the next day?

Do you feel unmotivated, irritable, low? *Do urges increase?*

Do you move your body daily or weekly? Monthly or rarely? How does your body usually feel?

◆

It's not an issue of being perfect in these areas—but of caring about them, possibly more than you have been, or, for some of you, of caring at all. I'll discuss the basics later in the guide. For now, I wanted to plant the seed.

Other Diagnoses

As I got older, aside from excoriation, I started dealing with other conditions and disorders.

BFRBs can be comorbid with (this simply means "present at the same time as") anxiety, depression, body dysmorphic disorder (BDD), substance use disorder, attention deficit hyperactivity disorder (ADHD), obsessive compulsive disorder (OCD), hoarding, self-harm, and more.

Like "BFRB," these labels are just a way to communicate about shared experiences so we can help each other overcome obstacles.

As of this writing, BFRBs are said to be "related" to OCD,[9] but they are not OCD in and of themselves. Also, BFRBs are not self-harm—you are not trying to hurt yourself with your BFRB.[10] However, some BFRBers have OCD or engage in intentional self-injury as well (comorbid).

Alongside healing your BFRB, learn or continue to learn how to manage other conditions or disorders you may have. Any strides will only help your picking, pulling, or biting. **The better you feel, the better you can manage your BFRB.**

My dermatillomania is unrecognizably better now, despite my issues (some of which I'm still dealing with). The help and resources are out there. Some are even listed at the end of this guide.

Treatments Are Effective

Just because you haven't been able to heal *yet* doesn't mean you can't.

Also, don't fall for "terminal uniqueness"—the belief that your version of something is unlike anyone else's, or that it's worse than everyone's so that, even though others may have been able to stop, you won't be able to. Otherwise, this thinking may be your downfall.

Even BFRBers with extreme cases recover.

No matter who you are, it's absolutely possible for you to stop. But first, you must *believe* that you can.

◆

If you're unfamiliar with treatments to heal body-focused repetitive behaviors and are still in the thick of it, you'll be pleasantly surprised by what you're about to learn.

When I decided in March 2019 to write this guide, I thought I had *discovered* how to solve dermatillomania and trichotillomania. If you've been a BFRBer for some time, you probably know not much information was out there in the past.

But as I got deeper than ever into the BFRB world, I learned my steps correlate with proven, existing, body-focused repetitive behavior treatments.

That said, these steps are presented differently, and though I've strengthened them with research for this guide, they're the same as when I first applied them myself: not medical or academic, but **approachable**.

◆

If you have come across therapies for BFRBs, please follow the BFRB Guide in earnest. Though all the information may not be new to you, I hope and believe you'll gain new insights and further healing.

The more we BFRBers engage with therapeutic content about this thing, the better.

The Steps

Step 1: Increase Your Awareness via a Log
Step 2: Identify Triggers and Keep a Thorough List
Step 3: Establish Protectors and Keep a Thorough List
Step 4: Practice Protectors

Step 1

Increase Your Awareness *via* **a Log**

Why Awareness Matters

Though you *know* what a BFRB is, this definition will be helpful:

> A BFRB is a deeply ingrained response to triggers that you may or may not be aware of.

I considered myself to be extremely self-aware. However, it turned out I wasn't nearly as self-aware as I thought, especially not when it came to my dermatillomania.

Tell me if this sounds familiar: One minute you promise yourself you won't pick and the next minute you find that you're doing it. This isn't because of a lack of commitment or desire. Very often, it comes from a lack of *awareness*.

Don't get me wrong. You may often be aware you're about to pick, yet the pull or nagging reminder (the **urge**) is too strong, so even though it's not a decision you want to make, you pick anyway.

Yet, I bet at other times you'll be picking for a while before you realize you don't quite remember when or how you started. Maybe you kind of do, but there's a gray spot in your memory.

If, looking back, you can't fully remember the moment you went from 0 to 60 (from not picking to picking), it could be that you do indeed lack awareness around your BFRB.

If you're like I was, you're not aware that you aren't aware, and none of this is sounding quite right. Once I shone a light on my excoriation, I couldn't believe how much of my picking had been clouded. But with increased awareness, I had taken the first step toward healing—as will you. By increasing your awareness, you'll begin to dismantle your BFRB.

Even if you have a good understanding of the details regarding your BFRB, I'm willing to bet it can deepen further, and it's important it does, so, please, follow along.

How to Increase Your Awareness

Maybe you've kept some sort of record before, like I have. I used to mark an *X* on my calendar every day I picked. My goal would be to not pick for the month, yet the calendar would be filled with *X*'s. I'd download sobriety and goal-tracking apps and modify them for my BFRB. But before long, I would stop keeping track of when I did or didn't pick. Recording my continued failure was demoralizing and useless.

Keeping a log, the way I explain below, is much more helpful. Its purpose won't be to hold you accountable or to encourage you to meet a streak (though it might).

As we've just covered, it's not enough to record *that* you've picked, so as part of the log, you'll not only log that you picked, you'll also answer a few questions each time you do.

> *If you've kept a BFRB log before, follow along anyway to find out where your log may have gone wrong (if you quit logging) and just how a log will start your healing.*

What You'll Log

If you scrape off a scab or pop one small pimple but then stop, you may not feel that's worth recording (though you absolutely can, and it'll be helpful if you do). What I most want you to log are the **sessions** (many call them **episodes**): the times when you pick more than a few tiny things, all the way up to engaging in a full-on massacre.

> *If you pick or pull continuously throughout the day, or do it in your sleep, this guide will still help you. Follow along with the log as best you can, and stay tuned for the upcoming steps.*

Before long, you'll know what makes a session for *you*—though it'll likely be when you feel like you "messed up."

That said, you don't have to wait to pick or pull to begin increasing your awareness. You can also log when you have a noticeable **urge** (anytime you've been fighting that pull, or nagging reminder, to engage in your BFRB).

Don't worry about logging every urge. That may be impossible. But please try to record most, if not all, sessions. If logging every session becomes too hard, log *at least once a day*.

For faster healing, log more, not less.

◆

While logs you can print exist, the following method allows you to start logging **right away**, whether or not you have access to a printer. By logging as recommended below, you'll soon know enough to be able to create your *own* logging method, if you'd like.

If you use a BFRB *app, and are enjoying it, this can be your log. That said, I find the below to be more complete and customizable, and thus likely to lead to more awareness. It also gives you as much or as little room as you need.*

Things will become perfectly clear as we go. For now, let's create your log so it'll be ready for you.

Creating Your Log

Before we continue, let me explain how important it is to log. Have you ever attended therapy, watched a video, or read a self-help book (on any topic or for any reason) and took in what you could without doing the work recommended by the author, therapist, or coach? You surely grew—but *not as much as you could've*. In this case, it might mean you reduce your picking but more or less remain stuck with your BFRB.

If you don't enjoy writing or journaling—this log doesn't have to be that. You can give short answers to the log's questions (I'll reveal what they are in just a moment).

Think about how much time you spend picking.

If you can pick for several minutes up to several hours, you can spare a few minutes to log in order to have the best skin, hair, or nails you've had in a long time or, possibly, in as long as you can remember.

Alternatively, you'll at least pull up these questions and ponder them (without typing or writing anything) when you've fallen into a session or are having a noticeable urge. This isn't as good at increasing your awareness, and I don't recommend it, but it is better than doing nothing.

In the end, it's up to you to take this first step toward healing your BFRB. This process—any process—only works when you participate.

Know that if you don't keep a log, you won't have truly followed the steps, and your healing may be limited.

◆

Here are the questions you'll soon be answering.

When you've picked, pulled, or chewed . . .

- Date?
- Time?
- How long did I engage for? (*How long?*)
- What was I doing before the session? (*Doing before?*)
- What was I feeling before? (*Felt before?*)
- What did I feel during? (*Felt during?*)
- What did I feel after? (*Felt after?*)

When you have an urge . . .

- Date?
- Time?
- What am I doing as this urge is surfacing? (*Doing what?*)
- How am I feeling? (*Feeling what?*)

◆

While I love notebooks and writing by hand, I log in a **note app**, which I access via my phone or laptop.

A pitfall with a physical notebook is that you may not keep up with the log if it isn't nearby when you need it, or if you misplace it. So, especially if you already take notes in an app and are comfortable doing that, I highly recommend using an app.

If you want to try a **notebook**, however, especially if you're used to writing by hand and enjoy it, please do.

> Note app or notebook—choose one and go for it. You won't know what works for you till you try, and it's no big deal to change your mind.

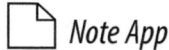 *Note App*

Open your note app of choice, and create a new note. Title it BFRB Log, or whatever you'd like. Then type the following questions. Leave them blank. *Please do this now.*

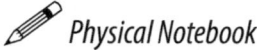 *Physical Notebook*

To continue with a notebook, please get one right now—I'll wait.

Do you have your notebook? Great. Jot the following questions on the first page. Leave them blank. *Please do this now.*

Below are the questions to copy into your note app or notebook.

DATE?

TIME? | HOW LONG?

DOING BEFORE?

FELT BEFORE?

FELT DURING?

FELT AFTER?

The above will apply when you just gave in to a **session** of picking, pulling, or biting. The following will apply when you have an **urge** but haven't picked.

In your **note app**, simply type the following questions below the first set.

 In your **physical notebook**, to save room for future questions, write the following on the next page.

    URGE

    DATE?

    TIME?

    DOING WHAT?

    FEELING WHAT?

◆

Please keep the questions more or less the same. Add questions if you'd like, but don't add so many that logging will be overwhelming.

An example of a question you *may* like to add to the first set of questions (the one meant for sessions):

- Where did I pick (or pull or bite)? (Shorthand can be *Areas?*)

◆

Have you typed, copied, or written the questions? Once you have, let's move on to just *how* to log.

For **Physical Notebook Instructions,**
skip ahead to page 41.

Keep reading for **Note App Instructions**.

How to Log Using a Note App

Assuming the note you just created is at hand, next to the note's name, type the month and year, e.g., **BFRB Log – April 2024**.

◆

From now on, when you log:

- COPY all corresponding questions from the top of the note and PASTE them below.
- Answer the questions.

For example, your log may look like this:

BFRB Log – April 2024

DATE?

TIME? | HOW LONG?

DOING BEFORE?

FELT BEFORE?

FELT DURING?

FELT AFTER?

URGE

DATE?

TIME?

DOING WHAT?

FEELING WHAT?

Keep these top questions blank for future copying & pasting.

DATE? **4/1**

TIME? | HOW LONG? **8 pm | 41 min.**

DOING BEFORE? *Answer*

FELT BEFORE? *Answer*

FELT DURING? *Answer*

FELT AFTER? *Answer*

> *After a BFRB session, this question block was copied from above and pasted below. Then the answers were typed in. For an urge, the urge questions would've been copied and pasted instead.*

If you have more than one BFRB, label the entries **Trich** or **Derma** or whatever resonates with you. For example:

DERMA

DATE? 4/1

. . .

TRICH

DATE? 4/1

. . .

◆

Next month, you'll create a new log note. It's easy, but feel free to bookmark this page or snap a picture of these instructions so you can reference them. You will:

- Open the latest log note and COPY the questions *from* the top.
- Open a new note and PASTE the questions *at* the top.
- Name the new note (e.g., BFRB Log – May 2024).

To easily find your current log, "pin" the note to the top if your note app allows it, or search for key words, such as "April" or "BFRB Log."

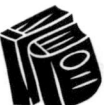

If you run out of space before the month is over (some note apps have a word-count limit), make another note. Create as many as you need and name them accordingly. For example:

- BFRB Log – May 2024 – **A**
- BFRB Log – May 2024 – **B**

◆

Working with your note app may take some finagling, but don't let that discourage you. Soon, it'll become second nature.

For organization, I get creative with capitalization, spacing, and symbols. You might do this and even give the note a color other than the default, for fun. (Little tweaks make life more enjoyable!)

Ultimately your log will and should reflect who *you* are and, especially at first, remain simple, to make it as easy as possible for you to log.

Skip to the thumbs-up to continue.

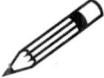

How to Log Using a Physical Notebook

Right now, write the current month and year (e.g., **April 2024**) at the top of the next fresh page.

◆

From now on, when you log, to avoid having to write the log questions over and over, flip to the front of your notebook and refer to the questions there. Flip back and forth as much as you need to.

Stay organized with **bullet points** as you go. For example:

April 2024

4/1   8 pm   41 min.

- *Answer to question 1*
- *Answer to question 2*
- . . .

If you have more than one BFRB, label the entries **Trich** or **Derma** or whatever resonates with you. And be sure to label an **Urge** as appropriate. For example:

April 2024

4/1   8 pm   41 min.   TRICH

- *Answer*
- *Answer*
- . . .

URGE   4/1   10 pm   DERMA

- *Answer*
- . . .

◆

Next month, you'll write the current month and year at the top of a fresh page and repeat.

◆

For organization and fun—draw, doodle, and add color as you see fit. (Little tweaks make life more enjoyable!) Ultimately, your log will reflect who *you* are. Especially at first, though, keep it simple to make getting into logging as easy as possible.

◆

Keep your notebook in a pocket, backpack, or purse to log on the go. At home, retrieve the notebook, log, and then put it back. Or, if you primarily pick at home, keep the notebook by your nightstand, on your desk, or in a drawer—wherever is most convenient.

Either way, put it back in its spot once you're done logging. *This is where the notebook lives.*

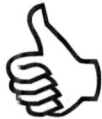

App or notebook, that's all you need to know.

Life will go on as usual, and the log will only come into play when you pick, pull, or bite, or during a noticeable, nagging urge.

Commit to Your Log

Ideally, you'll log right after a session. But in reality, sometimes you may be out and about or be unable to log right away for some other reason.

Log when you can. Do the best you can, and don't worry about it.

But commit.

When I started logging, it became so annoying that I would think, *Ugh, if I pick, I have to record it, so I won't pick*... Of course, I picked anyway, so no, these steps aren't about annoying you till you stop. (Ha!)

Don't use the idea of not counting tiny things as an excuse to pick or pull and *not log*. If you start to use it as an excuse, vow to log *everything*, or otherwise be consistent about what makes a session (e.g., two tiny things and up) and stay the course.

As you start logging, if you identify something that's making this process hard for you (such as where you place your notebook), adjust what you can to make it easier (e.g., move your notebook).

The easier you make this for yourself, the better. But once you see the evolution surrounding your BFRB, you'll need little encouragement to keep logging even when it is tedious. Soon, you'll start to see how incredibly helpful a log is.

What Logging Will Be Like

To be honest, my log is messy.

I write in it quickly. I use wording that wouldn't make sense to others but that resonates with me. I might go off-script and start asking and answering new questions (such as LESSON LEARNED?), because I've hit on something important or had an epiphany (hello, increased awareness!).

It's OK to have a messy log, as it's only meant to aid in BFRB healing.

Below I'll walk you through what answering the questions may be like so you'll feel fully comfortable when you start logging. The examples below have been modified from my own log.

Sessions

What Was I Doing Before the Session?

Write down what you were doing (e.g., studying or chores) and/or what you were *going to* do (e.g., study or do chores).

If you remember, in Why We Pick I explained that generally we pick to escape, so write anything you think you might be trying to escape.

For example:

Doing Before?
Was about to write to meet my daily novel word-count goal; scrutinized my face in the bedroom mirror. I just got up and did it.

◆

Though the point of the log is increased awareness—largely around what unwanted or uncomfortable things you may be trying to escape—sometimes no negative feelings or difficult tasks will be obvious. That's perfectly fine. As best you can, record what you were doing before that session.

Here are examples:

Doing Before?
Making lunch. Went to the bathroom to pee.

Doing Before?
Was watching a show on the couch. I started running my fingers over my skin, and then I began picking.

Doing Before?
I guess I was massaging my shoulders. That turned into me feeling texture on my skin and wanting to go see it in the mirror.

The goal is to increase awareness around *everything* you do before engaging in your BFRB—down to the smallest detail, and this includes your own movements and actions. These details are important, especially the ones that lead directly to your picking.

> As you log, identify whatever happens or is present, or whatever you do, think, or feel, right before your BFRB session.

What Was I Feeling Before the Session?

This will pertain to whatever you were doing or were about to do before a session and how you felt about it and/or how you felt in general.

Here's an example of how I'd answer this question at first:

Felt Before?
Fine.

Many of my entries looked like this for a while, but over time, I realized I could prod "Fine." Though, even when I knew "Fine" wasn't the full story, there were days I didn't have the insight to know what was really up. And every once in a while, "Fine" was the truth.

Sometimes you'll be inspired to think about the questions deeply. These thought-out recordings will be the most helpful. Other times you'll jot an entry and want to move on quickly, because you're angry or upset that you picked, or you have stuff to do. That's OK. Every entry is helpful.

Here are examples of answers that are a little more fleshed out, though:

Felt Before?
I wasn't looking forward to writing my novel, and it's stressing me out. I think I'm stressed because I'm unsure where to take my story.

Felt Before?
I keep thinking about that project. I should start it. Maybe I felt like I was putting the project off by watching the show.

Though some of the log questions are about what you're **feeling**—what you're **thinking** can be intertwined with that, so for this and any other question that asks about feeling, log any individual thoughts or trains of thought that you can pick out or remember too.

◆

All this said, don't worry about answering perfectly.
    Just log.
    All you have to do is answer each question down the line—nothing more.

What Did I Feel During the Session?

My reply to this question, especially at first, could look like this:

Felt During?
I dunno.

And as I *kept* logging, like this:

Felt During?
Focused, determined, consumed, lost, whirlwind.

Felt During?
Relaxed, focused.

When you try to answer what you felt during your BFRB session, you may face that gray spot I mentioned earlier and realize you don't know or don't remember. This is to be expected. With time, recalling will become easier.
    This question helps you explore not only what may be going on in your mind (specific thoughts and emotions) but also what positives your BFRB provides you (e.g., relaxation, time to think freely about a topic, entertainment).

Remember, picking or pulling is not only an escape route; it gives us some benefit once we've escaped.

What Did I Feel After the Session?

Your answer here can be long and cathartic, or depending on how you feel or how pressing the tasks you're doing are, it can be short, like this:

Felt After?
Mad. Quiet.

As you begin to heal, your relationship with your BFRB will change and so might your answers. Here's an example from my log after I had been following the steps for a while:

Felt After?
I feel as if I can stop picking, so now I don't really want to. Like . . . I can stop later.

Use this question to explore *whatever* you feel after a session. Try not to judge or "fix" these strange, nuanced, or complex thoughts or feelings. *Harness* what you learn instead.

For example, one skin picker identified the negative emotions she felt after picking and considered that maybe she picked to *purposely* feel that way, because, maybe, she got something out of it (the mind is capable of stranger things). So she chose to *not* feel regret and self-hatred after picking, when she could help it, so it wouldn't be an incentive.

At one point, I too chose to not give in to the crappy feelings, or at least to not sink into them as deeply as I had in the past. After all, post-picking frustration and anger had yet to heal my BFRB.

◆

This question also offers a chance to encourage yourself.

Felt After?
I'm happy I didn't pick at my back, chest, or face. I only picked at my legs. That's a win.

Time?

Some BFRBers tend to pick at around the same time of day. This has little to do with the clock; it's about what we're usually feeling, doing, or needing to do at around that time, which could be dictated by schedules and routines—studies, work, or family.

By recording in your log, you'll concretely learn what those recurring things are for you. An estimate of what time it was when you started is just fine.

How Long Did I Engage For?

What you write here can be exact, if you look at the clock before and after. For example:

Time? | How Long?
8:50 pm - 9:16 pm | 26 min.

However, your best guess is fine too:

How Long?
< 1 min.

The above—"less than one minute"—would apply to a short session, where maybe you got one or two things. Another example:

How Long?
10 min.-ish

◆

How long you pick or pull for can become a metric for tracking your improvement, but I ask you to not keep score yet. We'll save tracking your improvement for later.

Where Did I Pick (or Pull or Bite)?

Depending on your BFRB, this question may not be useful (if that's the case, don't include it). But if you're like I was—though your BFRB affects many areas, it's a *priority* to stop picking, pulling, or biting certain parts of your body. For that reason, seeing that you avoided a specific zone (e.g., face) can be useful for morale.

This is how I've answered this question before:

Areas?
Chest, shoulders, legs, back

Areas?
Face (minimal!), chest (pretty bad)

Areas?
Face, but I didn't go for things too roughly.

Noting the severity of your session, as above, can be helpful. For example, guilt can lessen when you realize you didn't do as much harm as you could've.

◆

If you do include this question, don't overthink it; and if you end up not finding it useful—cut it.

Urges

What Am I Doing as This Urge Is Surfacing?

Write what you're doing (e.g., getting into bed or finished showering) and/or what you're going to do (e.g., go to bed or shower) as this urge is surfacing.

How Am I Feeling as This Urge Is Surfacing?

Record how you feel about the current task, or your general mood.

Physical sensations can also be written here, since they offer clues as to what's going on with you as well. *How am I feeling?* can be interpreted many ways (emotional, physical)—cover as many bases as you can.

As above, consider what you're **thinking** about too, as this influences how you're feeling.

A Final Word on Step 1

Keeping a log isn't that fun, but it's great for making you very aware—not *kind of* aware—of the feelings, thoughts, situations, and actions surrounding your BFRB.

This is key.

Please, at a minimum, create your log (in a notebook or note app) before moving on.

When you experience increased awareness, you may better understand the following steps, so if you'd like, focus only on Step 1, on logging, for a few days to a week or so.

Set a reminder to return to the guide.

If you're on a roll, keep reading!

◆

A log is not how I intend for you to stop picking. Three steps remain. Let's go!

Step 2

Identify Triggers & Keep a Thorough List

What Are Triggers?

Picking, pulling, or biting doesn't spring up from nowhere. That is, you don't pick for no reason. A catalyst always exists. We call this a trigger.

You may remember the word "triggers" from our definition:

> A BFRB is a deeply ingrained response to *triggers* that you may or may not be aware of.

A **trigger** is whatever happens or is present (or whatever you do, think, or feel) that leads to a session. Since they precede sessions, I also call triggers precursors.

Though triggers are broad, you can think of them as *roughly* falling into three categories.

1. The Desire to Escape

Triggers are *usually* those things we use our BFRB to escape from: stress, aimlessness, nervousness, indecision, worry, guilt, boredom—*any* discomfort or distress, large or small. These are all triggers!

More specifically, these feelings (or sensations) are caused by things such as:

- Tasks and to-dos (e.g., work, studies, chores, writing, watching TV)
- People or events (e.g., a family member, a certain friend, an upcoming meeting)
- Our physical state (e.g., tired, hungry, achy, hot, cold)

The feeling and the thing that caused the feeling—*both* are triggers. We can also go deeper to discover more triggers.

For example:

- The *aspects* that are making a task or activity tough to do can be triggers.
- Wanting to talk about a disagreement with someone but worrying about their reaction can be a trigger (this is more to the point than singling out that entire person as a trigger).
- Feeling unprepared for a meeting, or even *more* specific, feeling like you didn't read up on the meeting topic sufficiently can be triggering (both are more to the point than just "work").
- Having just eaten too much junk can be a trigger, because it causes feelings of guilt or physical discomfort, or because whatever you were escaping via *snacking* is still there, asking to be fled from again—this time via picking or pulling.
- Not having a solid plan of what to do in the evening after work or homework, and thus feeling aimless, can be a trigger.

◆

To summarize, because they're different ways of viewing the same thing—i.e., whatever we're desiring to **escape**—all of these can be considered triggers.

2. Avenues of Escape

Above I said triggers are *usually* those things we use our BFRB to escape. What about the rest of the time?

Well, triggers are also avenues through which we *can* escape or things that are *related* to these avenues of escape.

This includes exposed skin; a blemish, pointy hair, or rough skin; seeing picking or pulling tools that are lying around; mirrors; as well as distinct reasons that bring us to these triggers (e.g., going pee, showering, and brow-tweezing bring us near the mirror).

> When faced with these triggers, we may pick even if we aren't particularly desiring to escape.
>
> For example, walking by a mirror or seeing a patch of exposed skin can have us scrutinizing and then picking, even if we feel

truly fine. This is because we're so used to doing this when we are pressed that it's easy to fall into in general. This is part of what I mean when I say BFRBs are a hardwired habit.

But usually and more importantly, we interact with these triggers (e.g., mirrors, exposed skin) as a way to **escape**.

Because it'll be useful to know where these triggers happen or are present, we'll call **locations**, e.g., bathroom, bed, desk, bedroom, car, triggers too.

3. Angling to Escape

When I'm not using the terms interchangeably, I make a distinction between triggers and precursors.

Precursors are the result of the triggers described above. They are those BFRB actions and movements that we do *seconds* before a session, as we're starting to seek a way out—an escape.

We're all familiar with these actions, which feel nearly impossible to backtrack from. They include:

- Running fingers over scalp, skin, or lashes
- Leaning into a mirror to scrutinize the skin
- Inspecting a spot or exposed skin
- Having a thought about target areas (e.g., *How is that blemish doing?*)

> As above, we may engage in precursors even if we aren't particularly desiring to escape. For example, despite feeling fine, we may have an itch and after scratching, our hand may keep mindlessly roaming in search of texture, since we're so used to searching for texture when we are pressed.

But usually we engage in precursors when angling to **escape**.

•

Don't overthink the categorization of triggers and precursors. Doing so won't help your healing. What's important to know is that **things lead you to pick and that you're capable of identifying what they are.**

Clear-cut categories and definitions aside, *notice* what you do, feel, think, or experience before you pick.

Why Identifying Triggers Matters

To understand why identifying triggers is powerful, think of precursors and triggers as signs.

Right now it's like you're on a bike, riding on autopilot. Hidden on the other side of some trees is a cliff, and you pedal right off, over and over. (Thankfully, in this metaphor, you magically regenerate.)

A trigger you've identified is a sign that says CLIFF AHEAD.

That thing you realized caused you to pick yesterday? How strange it will feel to see that today you're noticing it *before* picking, before riding off the cliff. As your triggers play out in front of you, you'll start seeing your dermatillomania with new eyes.

We're not at the final step, but by *noticing* the sign that you're about to pick (even if you notice it too late), you're closer to where you want to be.

How to Identify Your Triggers

You'll identify your triggers with the help of your log.

> *Though* BFRBers *have triggers in common, your life is brimming with ones that are unique to you. That's another reason logging is important.*

While logging a **session**, start from the moment of picking and work backward, calling up every link in the chain of events that led to it.

If logging an **urge**, consider what's happening right now that you may be craving to escape—whatever you might want to soothe, address, solve, etc. If that isn't giving you clues, think of what happened recently in your day, or throughout your day as a whole.

> *As your awareness grows, you'll be able to get more specific. But to start, identify the general feeling (e.g., stress) or the task or condition (e.g., homework) that's triggering you if that's all you can do.*

•

You must *know* your triggers.

Because identifying triggers and then forgetting them isn't helpful, you'll be keeping a list of them.

To go from healing someday to healing now, **you must do the work**—thankfully, this list is easy! Whether or not you've identified any triggers yet, let's create your list now so it's ready as soon as the next, or first, trigger is revealed.

Creating Your Triggers List

If you log in your note app, stick with that. If you use a notebook, you can switch to a note app, or keep writing by hand. Both approaches have their plusses and minuses, so choose what feels right. You can always change your mind later.

For **Physical Notebook Instructions,**
skip ahead to page 60.

Keep reading for **Note App Instructions.**

How to Keep a Triggers List in a Note App

Open your note app and create a new note. Title it Triggers, or whatever you'd like.

For a while, I simply listed my triggers as I noticed them:

TRIGGERS
- Item
- Item

Soon, I grouped related things and added headings (as best I could, given the broad nature of the feelings, thoughts, situations, actions, and tasks that come before a BFRB session). For example:

MANIA-MIND THOUGHTS
- Item

REASONS THAT BRING ME TO THE MIRROR
- Item
- Item

WORK-RELATED
- Item

Grouping items will help you get a feel for what your triggers *tend to be about*, and moving things around as you define categories will ingrain the items in your head, due to the repeated exposure, which will help you remember these triggers and thus be on the lookout for them.

But if you want to make things as easy as possible, start with a straight-forward list—if a messy one—and organize it from there only if you feel like it.

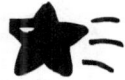

For fun and organization, add icons or symbols as bullet-points and consider giving this list a color other than the default.

Skip to the thumbs-up to continue.

How to Keep a Triggers List in a Physical Notebook

Open your notebook to the second section, which you can create now by placing a sticky note halfway into your notebook (the first half is the log).

Title the page Triggers, or whatever you'd like.

For a while, I simply listed my triggers as I noticed them:

Triggers

- Item

- Item

Before long, I grouped related things and added headings (as best I could, given the broad nature of the feelings, thoughts, situations, actions, and tasks that come before a BFRB session).

In a note app, I reorganize list items easily by copying & pasting. With a physical notebook, you'll have to get creative. One idea is to list triggers as they reveal themselves to you and then lightly shade them with different colored pencils (or different highlighters) as you make up categories for your triggers (such as Mania-Mind Thoughts, Reasons That Bring Me to the Mirror, Work-Related), i.e., each category gets a different color.

You can also designate symbols, e.g., a swirl, a triangle, a square, an eye, a star, to different categories.

Grouping items will help you get a feel for what your triggers *tend to be about* and, due to the repeated exposure, ingrain the items in your head, which will help you remember and thus be on the lookout for them. But if you want to make things as easy as possible, start with a straight-forward list—if a messy one—and organize it from there only if you feel like it.

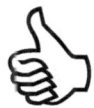

From now on, when a new trigger reveals itself, as you log or as you're going about your day, open up your Triggers List and add it, in whatever words ring true for you.

Feel free to ramble, ask yourself questions, write in shorthand, and let the typos flow. This is simply an aid in healing your BFRB.

If, as you list triggers and precursors, you have epiphanies about ways to address or ease them—**embrace this line of thinking**.

More Examples of Triggers

To bring this together, I've underlined the triggers in examples from Step 1.

Doing Before?
Was about to write... <u>scrutinized my face</u> in the bedroom <u>mirror</u>. I just got up and did it.

Felt Before?
I <u>wasn't looking forward to writing</u> my novel, and it's <u>stressing me out</u>. I think I'm stressed because <u>I'm unsure where to take my story</u>.

In this example, to escape the stress that surged while writing (*trigger*), I went to scrutinize my face (*precursor*) in the mirror (*trigger*), and then I picked.

Notice there's a chain of events: like dominoes, one trigger leads to another till you're picking.

These examples are from my own log, when I was at different levels of awareness. So some examples include **a)** what I wanted to escape, **b)** the avenues of escape I sought out, and **c)** how I angled to escape—the full chain of events—while others are limited.

Doing Before?
Making lunch. Went to the <u>bathroom</u> to pee.

This is bare. Still, we can find a trigger here. Being in the bathroom is a common trigger because as soon as some of us look down at our legs or pubic area while peeing, or lean into the mirror to scrutinize, we're likely to pick or pull.

Let me be clear about this:

The mirror is a *huge* trigger for many.

You may have already realized the mirror is a trigger, but note that each reason that brings you in front of it is a trigger too.

For example:

Doing Before?
I guess I was <u>massaging my shoulders</u>. That turned into me <u>feeling texture</u> on my skin and <u>wanting to go see it</u> in the <u>mirror</u>.

Here, what led to the mirror was wanting to see texture—different than going pee, yet both led right to the mirror. If being in the bathroom or in front of a mirror triggers you, you can never go to the bathroom or look at your reflection again. We'll discuss how in Step—

—I'm kidding. But stay tuned, because Step 3 discusses what we actually do with triggers.

For now, let's break down this next example. You may relate to this common scenario if you haven't related to the others.

Doing Before?
Was <u>watching a show</u> on the <u>couch</u>. I started <u>running my fingers over my skin</u>, and then I began picking.

Felt Before?
I keep thinking about that project. I should start it. Maybe I felt like I was <u>putting the project off</u> by watching the show.

While sometimes you *may* pick or pull in a situation like watching TV, massaging your shoulders, or going pee because it's become habitual, as you can see in this example, usually, with a little prying, something escape worthy, i.e., the discomfort or perhaps guilt of falling behind on a project, can be uncovered.

A Final Word on Step 2

If you haven't created your log, please do so right now. Make sure you've created your Triggers List as well. Then, please, take a moment to add any triggers or precursors you've already identified.

If you get ideas for how to ease or *prevent* your triggers and precursors, that's great!

However, for now, your main objective is to simply identify the things that come before your picking (even if strange, subtle, or embarrassing).

When you start noticing your triggers play out in your life, you'll better appreciate the upcoming steps, so if you'd like, continue logging and identifying triggers for a few days to a week or so.

Set a reminder to return to this guide.

If you're on a roll, keep reading.

◆

Identifying precursors to my picking was the catalyst in my healing—but that alone didn't do it.

The steps build on one another.

If you've followed the steps so far, be proud of yourself. Go ahead. Feel it. *Really.* Now, keep going.

Step 3

Establish Protectors & Keep a Thorough List

What Are Protectors?

You can probably relate:

Once you're at the edge of a session (staring down a blemish or curling your fingers around a hair), your chances of turning back are low, whether you want to or not. Or already in the middle of picking, pulling, or biting, you want to stop, but you literally can't.

Since stopping is so hard, *the key is to not start.*

Cue protectors.

By identifying your triggers, you're halfway there, because if triggers are one side of the equation, **protectors** are the other.

> Protectors counteract and prevent triggers.

By asking you to embrace ideas on how to ease triggers, I meant to get you thinking about protectors, but as we move through Steps 3 and 4, we'll explore them fully. That said, they can be simplified to being nothing more than what you can do to prevent a session. (Some can even help you exit sessions.)

I bet you've bumped into protectors in the past—BFRB "tips" learned along the way, or potential solutions you thought of yourself. These probably didn't help much, or they helped some but not enough.

In this step and the next, I'll explain mistakes BFRBers make with protectors and how to avoid them and, more importantly, how to apply protectors correctly, because once you understand protectors, you'll see they *are* the answer.

It makes sense that due to previous failure to stop, you may resist trying even simple protectors, and you may ignore big protectors because you believe they won't help and thus won't be worth the trouble. But I ask you to give all protectors a chance now that you're gaining deeper awareness of your BFRB. **Awareness is a key ingredient you were missing in your previous attempts to stop.**

While you may be familiar with some protectors, many will be new to you. You can think of protectors as *roughly* falling into three categories.

1. Foundational Habits

Foundational habits strengthen your foundation as a person. When this foundation is firm, it puts you in a position, physically, mentally, and emotionally to handle triggers and squash urges with relative ease.

By preventing the emotions and discomfort you want to escape, foundational habits also ***prevent* triggers and urges**—which means no picking or pulling. This is amazing for BFRB healing!

Since foundational habits cover a lot, let's break this category down. For most of us, foundational habits will fall into about six pillars:

1. The Basics
2. Relaxation
3. Tasks
4. Mindset
5. Personal Care
6. BFRB Targets

It makes sense to start with the basics since they form the very *base* of your foundation.

The Basics

Earlier I planted the seed of thinking about your basics, aka, how well and how much you **eat, sleep, and move**. If you're not operating well at a basic level, likely the rest of your life will malfunction.

Lazy, undisciplined, and unmotivated are what I thought I was. But it turns out I was often ignoring my most basic needs—I was sluggish, under or over fed, achy, or just tired (and hard on myself). To-dos seemed most troublesome then.

And my worst picking would happen.

Now I know why.

Bad *sleep* leads to lack of focus, making tasks more difficult and resulting in triggers. It also cuts into emotional bandwidth, again equaling triggers. *Eating* poorly leads to sluggishness, lack of motivation, difficulty concentrating, and thus the desire to escape via BFRBs as we're trying to go about our day. Meanwhile, if the body is achy and stiff due to lack of *movement*, that can compound with other triggers and have us using our BFRB to escape the discomfort.

Thus, anything that has you eating right, sleeping well, and moving some is a foundational habit. But don't stress if you have trouble with these areas (I certainly did and, sometimes, still do).

> Being healthy has lulls and highs—
> perfection isn't the goal. Striving to be
> good to yourself, over and over, is.

Here's an example of a foundational habit that isn't as big as overhauling your diet, but which still counts:

⚠ TRIGGER
Drinking too much coffee

🛡 FOUNDATIONAL HABIT
Set a limit of one cup of coffee per day.

Minimizing caffeine—which can lead to anxiety, physical discomfort, jitteriness, and thus roaming hands—is the protective habit. For some, the protector might be drinking zero coffee, if they're too sensitive to caffeine.

The thing about protectors is that they're *unique* to each of us. That said, under the upcoming section More Examples of Protectors, I touch upon foundational protectors that can get you started or move you further along.

> *This upcoming section will grow your understanding of your BFRB and fast-track your healing.*

Relaxation

Be it stress from work, to-dos, relationships, etc., even when I learned how big of a factor stress was in my life, I felt I didn't have time for **relaxation**.

Yet, I spent hours a week picking to de-stress and relax (even though I didn't know then that's what I was doing). Other ways we might force downtime is by eating junk food, scrolling social media, binge-watching shows, or binge-gaming.

Since we're going to force relaxation and de-stressing *anyway*, we're much better off if we take charge and purposely make time for moments of joy and calm, be it through:

- Reading a few poems.
- Going for a walk or run.
- Cuddling with a pet.
- Snacking on a bowl of berries.
- Getting comfy and watching a YouTube video, a movie, or one episode of a show—guilt-free.

Excess is what flips some of the above from beneficial to harmful. In moderation, they can be de-stressing and healthy.

If you're not used to regularly relaxing, you may not even know how you *like* to relax. Under More Examples of Protectors, I share plenty of activities you can try and explain *how they help against* BFRBs.

By the way, you can't relax one afternoon and be good for the month. Set aside time for meaningful relaxation and decompression every day (or most days). If that's not possible, do small things for yourself throughout the day and cherish them.

Relaxing before triggers and urges have even surfaced—so they have no reason to—is what makes relaxation a protective, foundational habit.

Tasks

While relaxing and minding the basics makes us more focused, happy, and willing when it comes time to perform tasks, eventually we just have to do them. And if you're anything like me, you're triggered while working, while studying, or when just *thinking* about starting in on something. I'm talking about all tasks and to-dos by the way.

Whether you're a student, employee, entrepreneur, home-maker, or creative, since **tasks** are a big part of our lives, wanting to escape them can have us picking or pulling *often*.

Thus, a protective foundational habit is:

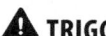 **TRIGGER**

Getting overwhelmed by large projects

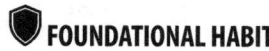 **FOUNDATIONAL HABIT**

Commit to working on a project for fifteen minutes to an hour to see how much you finish in that time. Use this info to estimate how long the whole thing will take and split it up into a certain number of pages or hours to complete per day.

Or **Brainstorm what the task will involve** and write out clear steps and to-dos.

Breaking every new project into manageable pieces, and laying out a clear direction and plan, is the foundational protector.

The point is to figure out how to make work, school, chores, passion projects, and life goals (e.g., writing a novel) easier to approach—less triggering.

Work that makes you miserable won't help your BFRB, though, so if you're sure you don't like what you're doing, by all means, up your life: make plans or moves to change your job or career. It's possible, with the right research, plan, and effort.

> You deserve to make a living doing
> something that makes you happy.

Regardless, you can manage whatever responsibilities you currently have to keep stress low and have fewer sessions.

Because they're essential for me to be BFRB-free, I'm a fan of productivity, organization, and time management—all protective foundational habits, some favorites of which I'll share later.

Mindset

For every emotion you feel like escaping via your BFRB, there's a lighter perspective. As I said earlier, thoughts can create feelings, and feelings influence thoughts.

But just because we land on unease, stress, anxiousness, worry, or *insert unpleasant emotion* habitually doesn't mean we have to *stay* there. We can develop a healthy and helpful **mindset** around work and projects, but also about ourselves, our relationships, our goals, our BFRB ... everything.

Here's a practical way to leverage mindset as a foundational habit:

⚠ TRIGGER

A tendency to feel stuck in some area of life

🛡 FOUNDATIONAL HABIT

Listen to affirmations at a set time of day, such as during your morning shower or drive to work, to get into a new headspace regarding some topic, or life in general.

> *This example shows the maintenance inherent in foundational habits. By weaving these habits into your day and your life, you improve both.*

Later, we'll explore the life-changing topic of mindset more.

Personal Care

Skin pickers can rejoice in knowing that time spent on the *right* **personal care** products, like exfoliants, will smooth skin by helping to eliminate and even prevent pimples, ingrowns, scabs, rough patches, and more.

Specific tips will be shared later, for hair, nails, and lips too, so you can see how pivotal this foundational habit is.

For now, understand that beauty and personal care routines are foundational because, by keeping pickable, pullable, and chewable targets to a minimum, *there are fewer things to tempt us in the first place*. For this reason, this pillar is related to the next and final one.

BFRB Targets

All can benefit from the above habits, but we're BFRBers, so at the end of the day, we have to live a little differently.

To avoid stirring up the compulsion, we must stay away from things we'll be tempted to pick, pull, or bite, aka, we must **avoid BFRB targets**. For example:

⚠ TRIGGER
Seeing or feeling a target and wanting to get it

🛡 FOUNDATIONAL HABITS

Scratch an itch with something other than your fingers in order to avoid feeling bumps, aka, potential targets.

Change the way you sit at your desk to keep from resting your chin in your hand, which can soon have you feeling for bumps on your face.

While washing your hands in the bathroom, make it a habit to have your eyes lowered, rather than staring in the mirror.

This is a clear counter: if seeing and feeling targets makes you pick, where possible, make it your new way of life to avoid touching or looking at target areas.

> *Depending on your BFRB, avoiding targets may be different. For example, it may be returning to a neutral mouth position. Throughout the rest of the guide, replace not looking and not touching with whatever applies to you.*

◆

Habits don't just exist; we encourage or stifle them.

Though this guide touches upon habit-building, its focus is on *which* habits are beneficial to heal your BFRB, and which to dissolve. At the end of the guide, I recommend a few books that cover habit-building and habits more in depth, as they're essential in all of this.

◆

Despite how important they are, foundational habits are not necessarily easy to build; eventually, though, they become part of you. However, because that takes time, and we don't always get foundational habits right, the next protector type—responsive habits—has our back.

2. Responsive Habits

Responsive habits are tailored to the moment. They're your best course of action once a trigger or urge *has* been stirred up. As the name states, they are a *response* to triggers or urges.

For every foundational habit, we find corresponding responsive habits, aka, ones related to the basics, relaxation, tasks, mindset, personal care, and BFRB targets.

Just because you didn't, or couldn't, prepare or nip this in the bud via foundational habits doesn't mean you can't still protect.

For example, if setting time apart daily for relaxation whether or not you're stressed, making you an overall happier, calmer person, is foundational, taking a break in the face of rising stress, right then and there, is responsive.

For example:

 TRIGGER

You feel frazzled, or down, and it's getting worse.

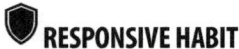 **RESPONSIVE HABIT**

Take a break. During the break, do an activity that gives you what you need. If you're overwhelmed, do something simple, such as drinking tea by a window. If you're feeling low, do something that lifts you up, such as dancing for one song.

Remember, the alternative is that you will likely force a break by picking, pulling, or biting. Taking a break is a different response to this trigger than engaging in your BFRB.

Another example of a responsive habit is putting a task off altogether for the rest of the day, if you can afford to at all. Suppose exhaustion or high stress is leading you to continually avoid a task and turn to picking—stepping back may be best.

That said, chronically avoiding difficulty leads us to pick as well, so reminding ourselves that we are capable and competent—that we can face all situations—is protective too.

In other words, if fostering a positive mindset by regularly listening to affirmations is foundational, countering anxious thoughts that are coming up due to a present situation is the responsive habit:

⚠ TRIGGER

You don't want to do a task, or attend an event, but you have to.

🛡 RESPONSIVE HABIT

Change your perspective. Consider why it's important to do this; remember that you're gaining experience that'll make you more capable and comfortable in the future; or consider whether this may be fun or rewarding with the right attitude.

◆

The goal isn't to *never* be triggered. To avoid triggers you'd need to find a bubble and never leave, which would become boring and unfulfilling, and, honestly, that may trigger you. (Ha!) The point is to be adaptive—responsive.

Since we can't get out of certain tasks, activities, or relationships (and often we don't want to), by figuring out the *specific aspect* of that thing that's troubling us, we get closer to practical protectors.

For me, this might look like this:

⚠ TRIGGER

Feeling unsure what to do next while writing

🛡 RESPONSIVE HABIT

Pause and open my note app or grab scrap paper to work through why. For example, I may find that even though this scene was in my outline, I no longer like it. From there, I may get more specific to see why I don't like it, or how I can change it.

Addressing the doubt, rather than stopping the novel-writing to pick, is the protective, responsive habit.

To reframe this so it applies to whatever *you* do:

⚠ TRIGGER
You don't want to do a task but you have to, or you want to, but it's becoming troublesome and difficult.

🛡 RESPONSIVE HABIT
Brainstorm obstacles (in your note app, on scrap paper, or in your head). Address these as best you can, or do whatever you need to do to lessen your resistance to it.

◆

Again, responsive habits are whatever you can, or need, to do in that moment to counteract a trigger/urge so you can keep from picking, pulling, or biting.

I won't go much deeper into this protector category here since I share many responsive habits in the upcoming More Examples of Protectors. However, I will highlight a special kind of responsive habit...

Go-To Actions

Responsive habits also counter precursors. As a refresher, **precursors** (not to be confused with protectors) are those BFRB actions and movements we do *seconds* before a session, usually due to looming triggers but sometimes out of pure habit.

For example:

⚠ PRECURSOR
Searching for pickable bumps after scratching an itch

🛡 RESPONSIVE HABIT
Pick up a small crystal to keep hands occupied, instead.

⚠ PRECURSOR
Leaning into a mirror to inspect skin

🛡 RESPONSIVE HABIT
Step way back and take a deep breath as you realize what you're doing.

⚠ PRECURSOR
Wrapping fingers around a piece of skin or a strand of hair

🛡 RESPONSIVE HABIT
Retract and snap your fingers as you realize what you're doing.

At the start of my healing, I'd feel tension in my chest, frustration, or even anger after I'd look away from my skin or the mirror, or retract from touching a target. I craved to look or touch, and yet I was keeping myself from it.

Instinctually, I'd take a deep breath to "discharge" this feeling.

This breath was my first go-to action.

A **go-to action** is a responsive habit that you do immediately after derailing a precursor, or stopping yourself from picking or pulling. It's a direct response to beginning your BFRB behavior. Since it's extra hard to just *not* pick or pull when you have so much momentum toward the cliffside, a go-to action gives you *something else* to do in that moment.

I'll offer many examples of go-tos and explain just how they work soon. For now, do *something else* right away when you've caught yourself beginning to engage in your BFRB.

Finally, be happy and congratulate yourself for choosing a new path.

> *I highly recommend you congratulate yourself after steering away from your BFRB, every time, if possible. This isn't just a nice thing to do; it encourages your brain to do it again next time. Just like the satisfaction from picking, pulling, or biting teaches us to do it again (for better or worse), celebrating each success trains us to keep protecting.*

◆

No one type of protector is the magic potion, just as no one type of trigger is wholly responsible for your picking. Yet, a mistake BFRBers make is attempting to stop by applying a smattering of protectors that address only a handful of triggers. They may focus on just a few foundational or responsive habits.

Because so many triggers are left out, this does little, contributing to the doubt that healing is possible.

I ask you to protect against every trigger you can—*all* the things you want to escape, the avenues you use to escape, and the ways in which you angle to escape (i.e., precursors).

> *This may not be possible all at once. But as you keep logging/identifying triggers, make it your **goal** to protect against every trigger.*

◆

Once I was more aware of my behavior, I could yank back against the tug to enter the bathroom and hang out in front of the mirror for no reason. But when I eventually had to go into the bathroom, I could get sucked into picking, despite knowing I should avoid looking at and touching targets.

You too may be sucked in despite your best efforts to keep away from targets. One way to make this easier is to add a level of physical protection. This brings us to the last protector type: barriers.

3. Protective Barriers

Barriers are not necessarily strong enough protectors on their own, but they should never be underestimated. To introduce them, here's a barrier I apply to this day:

⚠ **TRIGGER**

Being in the bathroom

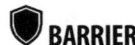 **BARRIER**

In the bathroom, I do not turn on the light; I use a night-light, or some dim light source.

> *Technically, dimness is the barrier.*

By blocking us from being able to easily look at or touch targets, barriers help keep the compulsion to pick or pull at bay. Other barriers include:

- Thin gloves
- Hats, bandanas, scarves, and wigs
- Long sleeve shirts, pants, and other protective clothing

By staying covered with these at home, and possibly at work, you can be more confident in your skin or hair when you selectively show it off.

- Band-Aids, placed on a pickable spot (e.g., blemish, scab, nail, finger) or on the fingers with which you pull (index or thumb)

You've probably tried barriers already. The thing is, even if certain barriers, like permanently covering mirrors, work for some, others are simply not going to keep up with them. Effective protectors are ones that are pleasant and convenient, or at least reasonable, for you.

I couldn't believe it when the simplest of barriers helped me manage this thing that had seemed impossible to control. I'm positive that you too will come to appreciate barriers that are a *fit for you*.

However, if you doubt a Band-Aid or a hat will help when you desperately want to pick or pull, you're right, it probably won't help.

Here are two reasons:

Soon is key.

In a way, barriers are responsive or foundational in and of themselves. And barriers are most useful if incorporated as foundational habits, aka, routinely and systematically—*long* before you're battling an urge.

Once we're speeding toward the edge of the cliff, it's much harder to turn back than if we stay far away from the cliff altogether.

For example, change into protective clothing in the morning, rather than because you've begun scanning your skin. Cover all blemishes right after washing your face or showering, rather than waiting till you're ruminating over a spot to make yourself choose between picking or getting up for a Band-Aid.

But suppose you forgot to apply a barrier, or you just need to apply one now, that's OK. Just do so right away. It can still help.

Still, there's something even more important when discussing why barriers may not work:

When things you want to escape grow and team up, that's when the desire to pick will surface and quickly intensify, and your barriers will go out the window. You'll start ripping off Band-Aids, flipping the light switch on, or yanking aside clothing to pick.

Trying to defy barriers is a warning to use to your advantage.

Ask yourself, *What's triggering me? What do I need right now?* Sometimes, it'll be obvious what you're angling to escape—do your best to address it.

Other times, you won't be sure.

But keep logging urges and sessions; you'll gain knowledge that you can use to brainstorm responsive and foundational habits to use *alongside* your wonderful, protective barriers.

Why Protectors Work

Every time we think a thought or do some action, we strengthen that thought or action's **neural pathway**, eventually creating habits, which are the brain's way of achieving efficiency.

Once neural pathways are "deeply ingrained," they become effortless—*no, compelling*—to travel down.

When it comes to BFRBs, and other destructive habits and behaviors, this efficiency backfires.

The neural pathways related to picking are deep and strong; this is why we pick so automatically—why it's so hard to stop once we've started. All the picking or chewing behind you has contributed to your neural pathways forging in a direction you don't want.

But neural pathways can be weakened, and strengthened.

The more we travel down the pathways of responsive and foundational habits, the stronger those become, and thus the less we travel down the pathways of picking, making these less ingrained.

For the last time, here's our definition from earlier:

> A BFRB is a deeply *ingrained* response to triggers.

Thanks to your awareness, you'll be able to see the CLIFF AHEAD sign (trigger) from a distance, so you'll have enough time and presence of mind to take a better path (protect).

Tamping down shrubs and unruly plants to forge new paths and habits will not always be easy (sometimes, it will be), but soon these paths will become wide and welcoming, while your pathways toward picking slowly but surely become overgrown, giving you pause before you embark down them, till, eventually, you don't bother to.

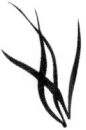

Neural pathways are the reason protectors are *not* an indefinite cop out, though it can seem as if some protectors—namely, barriers—are.

But if responsive habits are a new, better response to triggers, barriers pump the brakes and allow us the space to carry out those new responses. This is how barriers help us rewire and change.

As a bonus, protective foundational habits make it so we have *nothing to respond to in the first place.*

Earlier I said I would discuss a better way to deal. Healthier, more rewarding, or at least benign, protectors *are* that better way.

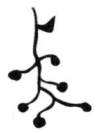

Don't let the mania mind convince you that getting hidden or small things is an exception. Doing so continues to wire you in the wrong direction—even if the effects aren't as visible. Not to mention, it may soon get out of hand and have you picking elsewhere.

◆

Before moving on, let's summarize:

It's possible to prevent triggers and urges from even happening. And now you know how: foundational habits like eating and sleeping well plus managing your responsibilities and mindset. This can mean getting eight hours of sleep, eating three nutritious meals a day, plus having a system for how you tackle your projects.

Next, if and when triggers and urges crop up, rather than defaulting to your behavior to cope, respond differently, with responsive habits. This can mean taking a break when you're stressed out, or even just being mindful when using the bathroom or scratching an itch.

Meanwhile, barriers, like covering target areas or keeping the lights dim, help you along the way.

Bottom line, whatever leads you to pick, you can counteract it with a protector.

How to Brainstorm Protectors

After picking, pulling, or biting, ask yourself:

- What could I have done to prevent this session?
- What can I do next time in the same situation?

Asking these types of questions is how you'll actively brainstorm protectors.

The log and Triggers List you set up in the previous steps will help you do this. Whatever protectors you come up with you'll carry over to a new list, which we'll create in a moment.

The process might go like this:

Log
Use your log to uncover what led to a session or urge. Once you have, write the triggers in your Triggers List.

Triggers List
As you're listing triggers, brainstorm protectors. After all, since protectors cancel out triggers, your Triggers List is a natural spot to brainstorm protectors. Once you've brainstormed something useful, carry it over to your Protectors List.

Protectors List
Your protectors go here.

> *You can brainstorm protectors in your log too. This process isn't meant to be rigid. Do what works for you.*

◆

Unlike your BFRB log and Triggers List, this new list will focus on the solution part (protectors) rather than on the problem part (triggers). In your Protectors List, you can also note overarching insights on your BFRB as a whole that you want to remember.

Establishing protectors as soon as possible will be the difference between beginning to heal asap or later, so let's create your list now to have it ready as soon as the next, or first, protector comes to mind.

Creating Your Protectors List

Follow my lead as you create this final list. Once you have the hang of it, you can log and list however works best for you (I touch upon variations at the end of the guide).

Do you have your notebook or device at hand? When you do, let's keep going!

For **Physical Notebook Instructions,**
skip ahead to page 86.

Keep reading for **Note App Instructions.**

How to Keep a Protectors List in a Note App

Create a new note. Name it Protectors, or whatever you'd like.

This can start out much like your Triggers List—as a simple list.

Even if you didn't create categories in your Triggers List, I do recommend you group related protectors and add headings or some sort of organization to this new list.

> *If you want, take a moment now to return to your Triggers List and capture any headings you may have inserted there that you can use here too.*

Another organization idea is to use the different protector categories (foundational habits, responsive habits, barriers) and their subtypes (the six foundational pillars, go-to actions) as headings.

Skip to the thumbs-up to continue.

How to Keep a Protectors List in a Physical Notebook

Flip your notebook to the back and start in from there. Title the page Protectors, or whatever you'd like.

This can start out much like your Triggers List—as a simple list.

Even if you didn't create categories in your Triggers List, I do recommend you group related protectors and add headings or some sort of organization here.

For example, if you assigned different colored pencils or highlighters (or symbols) to different types of triggers, use these for corresponding protectors (as best you can), or assign them now.

Another idea is to use the different protector types (foundational habits, responsive habits, barriers), to organize your list, by giving these headings to alternating pages, over and over.

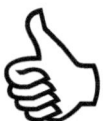

From now on, as you're logging and then listing triggers, brainstorm protectors too.

You don't need to include every single habit, good decision, or thought, but *most* protectors should make it in, no matter how small.

It may become tedious to carry items into various lists, but doing so will ingrain them in your head so you notice the warnings (triggers) and remember to heed them (protectors). This is true whether you rewrite the items in cleaner, more concise language—or just copy & paste.

To help you remember what your triggers are and how you can best protect from them, you can also skim your entire list each time you add a new item. Reorganizing your lists as you make up new categories will be helpful in this too.

I promise, this bit of effort will be more than worth it.

◆

At this point, try to identify triggers and brainstorm protectors every time you log. Try *something*—or brainstorm something to try next time—even if it's just your best guess.

To take out some of the guess work, though, read on.

More Examples of Protectors

I recommend you read most, if not all, of the following unless you can tell by the heading that it will not apply to your BFRB. In many cases, while it might seem like a protector is meant for a BFRB different from yours, you may find you can apply it. Many protectors help with multiple, different, body-focused repetitive behaviors.

Be extremely open to new tactics and even ones you've tried before—while confidently discarding ones that aren't for you (you can always come back and try things that don't interest you right now).

◆

I want you to have solid ideas as you keep logging, identifying triggers, and brainstorming protectors, so I'm about to offer many examples in this lengthy section. However, be sure to stick with it and tune in to **Step 4, Practice Protectors**, which will offer more crucial guidance.

To stay engaged as you read, keep doing the work, aka:

- List protectors you know will help you.
- List protectors you think *might* help you.

You'll probably identify triggers while reading the following sections too. Consider writing these in your Triggers List.

- Pause your reading to dig up a protector you want to start using.

- Pause your reading to adjust something in your physical environment.

Just be sure to not get distracted; then return to the reading.

◆

As soon as you browse the sections below, you'll be closer than ever to radically reducing your BFRB.

Let's keep going.

Relax, Unwind, Recharge, Decompress, Rejuvenate...

Relaxing, unwinding, recharging . . . it doesn't matter what you call it. Just make time to enjoy, play, do what you want to do, or just be. I know we're meant to feel joy—en*joy*—because when we go long enough without doing so, we get out of whack.

And nothing good comes from that, especially not for our skin, hair, or nails.

You may often feel high-strung, wound up, overwhelmed, frazzled, or tense before you pick, be it hours before or right before, but you may also feel burnt out, sad, or low. Either way, it's an indication that you need to balance out.

> High or low, when we're *out of balance* is when
> we're most prone to picking or pulling.

Stress may creep up on you throughout your day. When it does, de-stress as *soon* as possible. There's no need to get to the point that you're falling apart, or that triggers and urges have grown from light breezes to hurricane-force winds. Still, if you get there, even in the midst of strong winds, please attempt to de-stress via some *responsive habit*—this is a huge step up from picking, which, again, is what will likely happen if you do nothing.

If de-stressing from an "emergency" state, devote a good chunk of time to meaningful relaxation to truly get yourself into a different state.

Just as protective, if not more, is to incorporate relaxation routinely as a *foundational habit*. If you're going to *have* to relax to keep from your BFRB and other destructive behaviors, you might as well relax, beforehand, from good footing, rather than from the edge. This will elevate you higher and make you more resilient when you do face stress—rather than having you work overtime to stay at base level.

You can relax in the mornings, afternoons, and/or at night. (Many relax in the evenings after the day's responsibilities.)

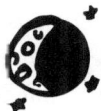

If you pick in your sleep, notice whether heightened picking correlates with stressful days and whether regularly relaxing helps.

♦

Referring to a list of pleasant activities is useful when out of balance, wanting a break, or looking to unwind. Feel free to create your own. Here are some ideas:

- Bathe or shower by candlelight. Possibly add salts, oils, petals, bubbles, or tea bags.
- Step outside barefoot or wearing thin socks to "ground" yourself (this practice is called **earthing**). If you're wearing shoes, touch a tree or a rooted plant (a house plant won't cut it here; the point is to connect to the earth).
- Open the door and look outside for a few.
- Color in a coloring book.
- Lie on grass. Possibly bring a blanket, novel, notebook, or laptop.
- With a candle or incense burning, draw or doodle. A wish or life ideal. Something that represents your life right now. Make up monsters. Worlds. Characters. It doesn't have to be amazing, or even good; throw it away or keep it.

- Pull tarot cards (draw just one or do a reading).
- Visualize being in a relaxing or exhilarating place. *You're swaying in the ocean, stalking through a jungle, lying in a field.*
- Sign up for a webinar or watch a live stream on a topic you enjoy. There are so many free ones, and often, these'll make you feel connected to others.
- Join a group (in-person or online).

Connection is healthy for humans (and you are one, I think), even if you consider yourself an introvert, as I do. So reach out to others. Your presence and connection brings value to them too. At the end of the guide, I offer resources where you can connect with other BFRBers.

- Attend a live or virtual event, such as a monthly open mic. Commit to being a supporter and make it to each one.
- Call a friend, cousin, aunt, uncle, sibling, godmother, etc. (actual call is better, but texts work).
- Pull up weeds (stress-relieving and entertaining, like hair-pulling!).
- Read through one or two email newsletters about topics you enjoy.
- Crawl into the covers with a mug of tea and just be (with no screens). This can be part of your night-time routine or done anytime you need to de-stress.
- Play Tetris, or another game, for fifteen minutes.

A BFRB session can be like a game—seek and destroy, one target after another. This is entertaining (stress-relieving), but so is finding a game you enjoy and allowing yourself to play it regularly, or when you need a break.

You know what your list doesn't need? Activities you'd *like* to enjoy, or think you *should*, but don't (look, coloring books aren't for everyone, but... maybe they *are* for you).

Also, be sure to write the things you *know* make you feel good, even if you don't do them as often as you'd like, yet.

♦

Because your neural pathways are eager to take those well-traveled roads of picking and possibly other destructive behaviors (e.g., binging), it may be hard to choose to balance out in healthier ways.

But it'll come more and more easily. You'll cherish the time in which you relax, regroup, refresh, decompress, unwind, recharge...

Below I go into more ways to rejuvenate that are particularly helpful for countering picking, pulling, and biting.

Get into the Moment

When we're in the moment, thoughts dissipate, and we feel that wonderful sensation of being *here*. But "being in the moment" is something you only understand once you experience it.

Though this is just one way to do it, what finally allowed me to "get out of my head" and into the moment on command was to tune in to my senses. The 5-4-3-2-1 Grounding Technique helps with this. So you see that it works, try it right now. Identify...

5 things you can see

4 things you can hear

3 things you can touch

2 things you can smell

1 thing you can taste

Don't worry about whether the things you focus on are worthy—just choose something.

♦

Other grounding techniques include tracing the outline of some object, like a door, or looking at an object, like a knickknack, in detail, really noticing its attributes (e.g., color, texture, patterns).

These techniques are a form of **mindfulness**.

> Put simply, mindfulness is being aware, present, without judgment.

◆

As a *responsive habit*, ground yourself when you need to balance out. Though tuning in to the present is satisfying anytime, many call up grounding techniques during moments of distress, such as panic attacks.

Additionally, if you feel you're being sucked into a session, or if you managed to exit one, you can tune in to your senses at that very moment, as a **go-to action**. This can make the switch easier by giving you something *else* to do and even dissipating some tension at not having allowed yourself to partake in your BFRB.

As a protective *foundational habit*, practice being mindful anytime you remember while doing the activities that make up your day, such as cooking, getting dressed, pouring tea, or working. Notice the auditory, sensory, visual, tactile, and olfactory experiences around you.

Meditate

Meditation is cited by many BFRBers as an incredible aid in their recovery. Even if you aren't drawn to meditating (though I recommend trying it), knowing why it works for BFRBers can guide you toward your own, similar, protectors.

Meditating is a lot like picking. As we meditate, we **focus**, just as we do while picking (namely in those trance-like episodes).

When we put all our attention on one hair, blemish, or scab—we exclude all else, and that means we remove anything and everything we craved to escape, e.g., overwhelm, pressure, worries.

Put differently, by zeroing in on one thing, everything else ceases to exist. This makes the world manageable, whereas before we found it not to be.

◆

When I thought it was "clearing your mind," meditating seemed nearly impossible. Once I realized it can look many ways, meditating itself became easy. Then, getting myself to do it regularly was hard. But I learned even that's easy.

To make meditating approachable, choose a designated spot (e.g., a certain rug, couch, chair, corner, window) as well as a time of day or day of the week and try:

Guided Meditation

Download a meditation app (Medito and Insight Timer are free), or type "guided meditation" into YouTube. Try a few videos till you find one *you* vibe with. Subscribe to a channel as a first step.

Labeling

After getting into your meditation position, observe your thoughts, and "label" them. One word, in passing, is all it takes, and you don't have to worry about getting it perfect.

Some label examples:

- Anger
- Frustration
- Remembering
- Planning
- Wondering
- Appreciating
- Analyzing
- Justifying

Don't judge your thoughts—just observe them—label them, send them off, and repeat. Enjoy the clear-headedness this brings.

Tuning In to Your Senses

For a few minutes, eyes open or closed, right where you are, tune in to some constant sound (such as a fan). Easy, right?

This is just one way you can tune in to your senses (in this case, hearing) to reach a meditative state.

◆

Done regularly, meditation can be a protective *foundational habit*. For example, you might set aside a chunk of time for it every Tuesday and Thursday or a small amount daily, e.g., just **three to five minutes** after work. Remember to have a designated spot for it.

Meditating can also be a *responsive habit*. Let me set the scene: You feel stressed and overwhelmed; you're starting to break down, so you drop everything and meditate for a few.

And if you have resistance to meditating...

Do Nothing

However you do it, you're up to the task of... no task at all. Doing nothing isn't necessarily meditating, though it can look like it.

I tend to lie on my rug, couch, or bed and set a timer for however long feels appropriate that day (e.g., three, eight, fifteen, twenty-five minutes), and I do nothing except be present and calmly take in my surroundings.

The Dutch have a word for doing nothing: *niksen*. Though in this Dutch concept, presence isn't a caveat.[1] Letting the mind wander into imaginative ruminations is fine, if not encouraged. Remember being a kid and looking up at the moon? Looking out classroom windows and day-dreaming? It's like that. And sometimes it's just what you need to do for yourself, though you may instead prefer to...

Create Space to Think

As we pick, our minds *replay or ponder problems and situations*, from a safe distance. (This isn't true for everyone, but it's true for many, especially in those picking trances.)

This rumination time is a benefit we may not realize we get from our behavior. Regardless, we can get it in a better way by creating time to *just think*.

Activities already discussed (e.g., coloring) can be moments in which to think and process. More examples include while:

- Brushing teeth or showering
- Walking outside or on a treadmill
- Cooking dinner or baking
- Eating breakfast

Because the body, and part of the mind, is occupied during these activities, you can think "at a safe distance" while you do these too.

◆

You might not decide "OK, I'm going to think now," but you can create easy, open, likely *silent*, moments in which to reflect on, process, and contemplate the day, what's come to pass, and what's underway.

Tap

EFT (Emotional Freedom Technique) or "tapping" involves using your fingertips to tap on points of the body in a sequence, while saying phrases related to the matter at hand, in this case a BFRB urge or a triggering situation.

If you've heard of it and have been curious, or if later on, you could use more protectors for balancing out, delve into EFT.

Be Grateful

Do you create gratitude lists already? Sometimes it seems like everybody does. Among benefits like a longer life, practicing gratitude releases dopamine and serotonin, decreasing depression and increasing happiness[2]—this is why gratitude lists are so popular.

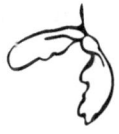

If you've heard of some of these potential protectors (e.g., meditation, mindfulness, gratitude) over and over and you haven't tried them at all, or in earnest—this is your time. Do it for your BFRB.

Your gratitude can be related to something you're stressed out about, or it can be about something completely separate. You can list two, six, or twenty items. Choose something significant, or tiny (a color, the incredible functions of your body, a song, something someone said, or a single sound).

Feeling positive about any aspect of your life will give a glow to every other area, while feeling negative about some aspect will bring forth the worst about every other area. This is how bad and good moods grow.

When you want to feel better, and you're unsure what to do, list things you're grateful for, and see some of your heaviness lift. This is a *responsive habit*.

To create a *foundational habit*, practice gratitude every morning, or every evening, in a list, or in your head.

As you practice gratitude, it'll weave itself into your everyday attitude, and you'll bounce back from problems more easily, resulting in fewer emotional triggers that push you to escape via your BFRB.

◆

Try it now so you can see what I'm talking about: What are three things you're grateful for right now? Don't overthink it; just be sure you're actually grateful—otherwise choose something else.

> *The idea isn't that gratitude alone will solve your BFRB. Remember, no one protector can. But the more tools you have in your toolbox to protect against emotional triggers, the better.*

Ask, What's Good?

Did you think of three things you're grateful for?

Seriously, try it.

But if gratitude isn't for you, or if you want a different take, ask yourself, What's good?

You don't like this about your looks. But what do you like? What's good?

You don't like this about your relationship. But what do you like?

You messed up there. But where did you do well?

Today, this went bad today. But what went well?

When something is bothering you, ask, What's good about this? as a *responsive habit*. Feel free to actually list it out. As a *foundational habit*, create a list like this regularly, *or* simply pay attention to the good throughout your day.

Journal

Because of the resilience and sanity it's given me, I've always been a fan of journaling. If you already journal, stay tuned for new ideas. If you've ever been interested or have dabbled but never stuck with it, read on for easy ways to start.

Before we continue, know that the goal is to express yourself openly—without judgment from yourself, and without thought toward *others'* input in some imaginary realm where they can see your thoughts as you write them.

And, certainly, if you're afraid someone will *actually* read your journal, keep it hidden (e.g., tucked discreetly in a closet). Otherwise, leave it somewhere convenient, such as your nightstand.

> *There may come a time where you want to write about something that feels too embarrassing or shameful—write it out anyway. Rip up and toss the page after if you need, or delete the entry.*

Journaling can be as easy as . . .

Write Whatever Comes to Mind

No filter, no judgment, no rhyme or reason: get wacky, get existential.

> *To make it even faster and easier, use a single word, phrase, or name to represent the whole. Aka, call, late, fight, mom.*

Write to Satisfy a Specific Need

For example, if you need confidence that day, write an entry that amps you up. If you need resolution, write out the problem followed by potential solutions or mindset adjustments. If you need closure, ideas, clarity . . . whatever it is, journal it out.

Create Lists

Lists are *very* low-effort, and effective. Ideas include a gratitude list, a dump of current worries or stressors, a list of areas in which you're confident or things you like about yourself, or a two-column list of the "roses" (the highlights of the day) and "thorns" (the trouble spots of the day).

Write About Your BFRB

Note moments of progress or enlightenment, and explore obstacles.

> *I used to frequently journal about picking after a session, distraught. Venting is a perfect use for a journal, but consider also using your journal as another place to increase your awareness, identify triggers, and brainstorm protectors.*

Refer to Prompts

I do this when I'm unsure what to journal, or feel resistance to it, but know it'll be good for me to do. Here are a few items borrowed from prompts I taped to my journal's front cover:

- Reframe worries over the coming day, or otherwise embrace the coming day.
- List two things you did well.
- List two things you're grateful for.

> *More often than not, I seal my entries with positivity or a silver lining (e.g., a bit of gratitude or encouragement).*

The Five-Minute Journal and others have prompts and space built in for your answers. If curious, look into them.

Though as a *foundational habit*, journaling daily, or almost daily, is an option, many benefit from journaling weekly, or even quarterly. For example, every quarter of the year, I write a long entry where I assess how far or near I am from my goals, note how I've been doing with my foundation, and record major life changes. I see where I'm going and where I've been, which helps keep me grounded and oriented in the right direction. (I set a calendar reminder to do this.)

Alternatively, you could use journaling to satisfy a specific need as a *responsive habit* when faced with a trigger, aka, drop what you're doing to journal.

A physical journal, a note app, or a digital journal, like Goodnight Journal, which you can access on any device, is an option.

Express Your Stress or Else

I came up with this saying for myself: "Express your stress or else." The "or else" was that I'd pick. If you give yourself no other outlet, you too may express your stress by picking or pulling.

Journaling (see above) is how I usually express my stress. For you, it may look like asking a friend or family member whether you can vent for a few, going for a run, or singing.

As a *responsive habit*, express your stress at times like these:

- In the middle of the work day, if stress is building and making you want to escape
- After socializing, shopping, or running errands

    Even after mostly positive interactions, or only a few fumbles—seemingly unworthy of addressing—we may still be over-stimulated, but we can decompress to neutralize this.

- Anytime you feel out of sorts

As a *foundational habit*, I express my stress at about the same time most evenings. If I don't have much stress to express, this may just look like **checking in** with myself.

Times you too might express your stress or check in regularly include:

- After work/school
- Before or after creative work
- Before bed

If you pick in your sleep, or have trouble sleeping, dumping worries in a journal at night may be particularly helpful.

◆

Regardless of what you do to express your stress, I recommend you choose *something*, since **expressing stress as often as possible helps keep triggers from bubbling over into a session.**

◆

Many of the items in nearby sections can be ways to express your stress, while some of them can be done *after* you've expressed your stress—aka, once you've poured out the bad, fill up with something good.

Checking in, expressing your stress, relaxing—all are related; sometimes they're the same thing. By trying them out, you'll come to know what's best for you, and when.

Breathe

I was never one for taking deep breaths at a moment of anger or stress. I don't know that I ever made it past one breath before deciding it wasn't working. After starting these steps and seeing how small efforts pay off, deep breathing has become a favorite protector.

Negative emotions impact our breathing, making us breathe shallowly. By purposely breathing deeply and slowly, we counter stress, anxiety, and more.

Deep breathing is not only extremely effective[3] but also readily available: the breath is a protector we carry with us.

Some breathing basics:

- **Have a straight spine**, whether sitting or standing, to achieve a full breath.
- **"Drop" your diaphragm**, the muscle beneath the lungs, as you breathe.

This dropping of the diaphragm is important, as it soothes the nervous system, bringing calm. Some imagine filling a balloon in their bellies or breathing all the way down to their feet. It can take a little practice to feel that drop.

- **Breathe in through the *nose* and out through the *nose*** unless a specific breathing exercise asks you to exhale through the mouth.

Now that you know the basics, here are three easy breathing exercises.

1

2:1 Technique

Breathe in through your nose for a count (e.g., four) and breathe out for twice as long (e.g., eight). Don't stop at the top or bottom of the breath—let the exhale roll into the inhale.

Try it right now.

Breathe in for 1 ... 2 ... 3 ... 4.

Exhale for 1 ... 2 ... 3 ... 4 ... 5 ... 6 ... 7 ... 8.

Do it again. Remember to drop your diaphragm and straighten your back. Do it once more.

Your count will depend on how fast or slow you go as well as lung capacity.

2

Alternate Nostril Breathing
*(aka **nadi shodhana pranayama**, which means "channel cleaning or purifying breathing technique")*

Block one of your nostrils with your thumb and inhale through the other. Now block the free nostril with your ring or pinkie finger. Exhale. Then inhale through this free nostril. Block it, and exhale. Then inhale through this free nostril.

Switch. Repeat.

This is just one variation of this breath. Try it three to five times in a row.

> *With breathing exercises, one breath may not do much. Two starts a change. But three brings it home. And more is better.*

3

Box Breathing

Breathe in through your nose for a count (e.g., five), hold for the same count, breathe out, and hold again.

Try it right now.

Breathe in for 1 ... 2 ... 3 ... 4 ... 5.
Hold for 1 ... 2 ... 3 ... 4 ... 5.
Exhale for 1 ... 2 ... 3 ... 4 ... 5.
Hold for 1 ... 2 ... 3 ... 4 ... 5.

And repeat a few more times.

♦

Assuming you followed along, choose the breathing technique you like best and call it up to change your breath during triggering moments as a *responsive habit,* or as part of your rejuvenation time as a *foundational habit.*

If nothing else, take a deep breath in and then exhale completely when you need to balance out.

Deep breathing and the following protector (which I love and practice daily) go hand in hand.

Practice Adhi Mudra

Cradle one or both thumbs with the rest of your fingers—gently, as if you're supporting or taking care of yourself.

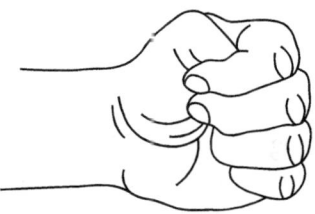

Some may know this as adhi mudra, a yogic pose, known to soothe the nervous system. Aside from bringing comfort, it's amazing for BFRBs because, in this position, you're "safe" from your BFRB: you know where your hands are; you're in control of them; you can't pick or pull.

Try it.

Hold your hands like this for at least three breaths. Spine straight. In through the nose... *fill the belly, drop the diaphragm*... out through the nose... Feel the change.

◆

Hold adhi mudra before entering situations in which you're used to engaging in your BFRB, such as sitting on the toilet. (This is *foundational*, and proactive!)

You can also do adhi mudra when you catch yourself engaging in precursors, or after diverting from picking or pulling. In other words, adhi mudra is a **go-to action**. For example, bring your hands down from your face or scalp, and then cradle your thumb in adhi mudra to give yourself and your neural pathways something other than picking or pulling.

> *If you enjoy adhi mudra, look into other yoga hand gestures, or "mudras."*

◆

The first few times you try the de-stressing activities listed here you might find them bland. Give them a real chance, though, lest you miss out on that life-altering try that has you understanding why recovered BFRBers swear by these things. However, if you decide something really isn't for you, that's OK.

Manage Sensory Input

Uncomfortable lighting, loud sounds, a temp that's too warm or chilly—manage your sensory input throughout the day so environmental stressors don't team up, especially with emotional triggers, and have you escaping the discomfort via your BFRB.

Here are some ideas:

Sight

Dim, brighten, or balance the lighting (in your surroundings and your devices), or take a break from screens, if your eyes are uncomfortable. If you've been looking at something close up for a while, look at something twenty feet away for twenty seconds.

Sound

Wear earplugs, earbuds, or noise-canceling headphones; walk away from or change loud or distracting sounds.

> *Alone, these simple changes won't affect your BFRB much. But combined with other tools, now that you have a greater understanding of your picking or pulling, they'll change a lot.*

Smell

Trade out conventional candles and air fresheners, if these bother you. Try more natural, softer options, or move away from overwhelming scents by going into another room or area.

Taste

Brush or floss your teeth. Drink something.

Touch

Get a sweater or fan; sip a cool or warm drink. Change out of irritating or uncomfortable clothing.

◆

Internally and externally—emotionally and physically—BFRBers can be more sensitive than the average person. I'm mentioning this only so you become more aware of sensitivities—so you do what you need to do to protect, problem-solve, and care for yourself.

> *While it can be annoying, heightened sensitivity can lead to great things, such as better art and more empathy. It's not always a bad thing. In fact, many see it as a strength.*

Stimulate Your Senses

I've mentioned tuning in to and managing your senses. Actively stimulating them is another protector.

While we can engage helpful thoughts and relaxation techniques, we can also balance out via the senses. For some, this works better.[4]

It's OK to stimulate or soothe yourself. However, to do it in ways that aren't picking, pulling, or chewing, try:

Sight

Stare into a crystal. Look at the sky, at a nice image/picture, or at a pleasant area of your environment.

Sound

Plug your ears to hear your heartbeat. Listen to whatever music you truly feel like listening to at that moment. Tap two crystals together.

Smell

Burn incense. Diffuse or sniff essential oils. Put your nose in a mint plant (these are easy to maintain!).

Taste

Chew flavored toothpicks. Suck on a mint, flatten gum against your palate, or nibble on a mint leaf. Munch fennel seeds one by one.

> *The tiny fennel seed is said to curb appetite and freshen the breath. Pick them up at any spice aisle. Chewing fennel seeds while working at my desk when I have excess energy is a protector of mine.*

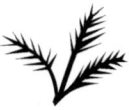

> *Switch things up if you find yourself getting bored; become a gum, mint, or spice enthusiast.*

Touch

Brush your arms with a soft brush over and over. Run an artist's paintbrush across your lips. Make knots in floss or fishing wire and run it along fingers or lips, feeling the bumps. Caress your skin, hair, nails, *or some nearby material*, in a non-triggering way. Chew on a sensory chew toy.

> *Especially if you chew, look into chew toys. Start with a soft one and trade off chewing with either side so as to not create imbalances.*

What you like about your behavior can guide you in choosing sensory protectors. For example, those who run strands of hair across their lips tend to enjoy running a paintbrush or silicone brush over their lips.

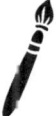

Personally, I enjoy the bumpiness of target areas (*touch*), as well as analyzing a blemish (*sight*), even hearing the slight pop (*sound*) when I pick. For these reasons, feeling the knots in dental floss (*touch*), staring into a crystal (*sight*), and tapping crystals (*sound*) are nicely stimulating to me. That said, I stimulate my other senses as well.

If you're not sure what mimics your BFRB, don't worry about it; just experiment. Add items to your grocery list (e.g., fennel seeds, brush) that interest you.

•

Keep items used to stimulate your senses near picking or pulling **locations** (desk, car, nightstand, coffee table). You can stimulate your senses while you work, study, drive, or relax as a *foundational habit*, to keep urges at bay in the first place. Or you can do it as a *responsive habit*, in response to some trigger.

Stimulating your senses is another great **go-to action**, giving you something else to do once you've stopped yourself from picking or pulling, or from rubbing a spot or scanning your skin in preparation to pick or pull.

Hand-Held

If you use your hands for your behavior, keep some protective object at hand.

A **hand-held protector** not only makes it so fingers aren't free to pick or pull, but also provides ways to stimulate a few of your senses (discussed above). It must be something you're happy to have in hand, though. To find out what that is, experiment.

Consider:

- A worry stone, crystal, rock, or seashell
- Stress balls, gummy or plastic sensory toys, putty (or things that are like putty—like silicone ear plugs)
- Bubble wrap (the good kind; some types don't pop well)
- Jewelry or spiral hair ties
- Acupressure rings

Finger pickers especially may want to give these inexpensive rings a shot—look them up!

- Scrap paper—which can be torn into a pile or folded
- A large coin or yo-yo
- Chinese medicine balls
- A fidget cube, or other fidget toys

Again, with your new awareness, BFRB "tips" you've heard about or tried before—possibly this one—can now help you.

◆

An example of how this works in real life: I keep a stone on my desk and pick it up when I'm reading something on my screen (when my hands would otherwise be idle). I feel any grooves or imperfections in it; I simply hold it, feeling the weight of it; or I rub the stone on my chest or shoulders, so that I'm soothing myself but not feeling any texture on these areas.

◆

Get into the habit of grabbing hand-held protectors even before your hands start roaming, as a *foundational habit*. (Whenever possible, be proactive.) You can also grab a hand-held protector when triggered, as a *responsive habit*.

If you've forgotten protectors all the way up to the cliff's edge, it's still not too late: grab some object right after you've diverted from your BFRB or precursors, as a **go-to action**.

In the Car

If you pick or pull in the car, I encourage you to keep those hand-held protectors we discussed in the cup holders and compartments.

Ideally, you'll grab these before your hands even start scanning, right when you get in the car, as a *foundational habit*. But if you don't feel like doing this every time, then certainly as a *responsive habit*, on days in which stress or anxiety are looming, or once you're already triggered, or as a go-to action when already starting to pick or pull.

Protectors specific to the car include:

- Install a fuzzy or textured steering wheel cover you can play with instead of pick.
- If you're the driver, position the rearview mirror as far as safety allows so you don't start to examine yourself in it.
- Keep a sweater or shawl in the car. Suppose you're wearing a tank top. In public, you may not pick, but in the privacy of your car, you may.
- In colder weather, wear gloves, as a barrier.
- During moments of stress, call up protective thoughts. You can't journal or express your stress in too many ways in the car, but you can still address triggers via your mindset.

Adjust Your Position

Adjust your body when you notice that your position is prompting you to pick. Triggering positions include:

- Resting your chin on your hand
- Propping your elbow on your desk
- Propping your elbow against the car door
- Propping your foot on your chair/couch

Start to notice which positions prompt you to pick and which don't.

This small habit of adjusting your
position makes a huge difference!

Mirrors

For so many, mirrors are *the* trigger.

Looking in the mirror when getting ready is one thing. Staring because we *happen* to be near one is a no for those of us with dermatillomania. In this section we'll cover both scenarios. Apply the following asap, to see an immediate reduction in your picking.

Remove Excess Mirrors

Get rid of excess mirrors, such as mirrors that are only for decoration, to the extent possible (I understand family, roommates, or landlords can get in the way of this).

Move Decorative Mirrors

If you'd like to keep them, decorative mirrors can be placed high on walls or behind deep furniture that prevents you from getting close.

Modify Decorative Mirrors

Modifying works well for mirrored sliding doors (which aren't easy to take down or replace) and for mirrors that you don't *want* to remove because, for example, they provide wanted brightness.

One skin picker makes sure her decorative mirrors have that fogged vintage finish that's hard to see in. Replace current mirrors with ones that are already altered, or look for DIY tutorials to modify the ones you own. Peel-and-stick sheets that mimic stained glass and the like can also be placed over mirrors.

If you can't modify mirrors in common spaces, modify as many as possible *in your own spaces*, or . . .

Manage the Lighting Around Mirrors

Protect against mirrors by dimming or changing the lighting around them. Here are some ideas:

- Use the hallway light and leave the door open when using the bathroom, if possible.
- Turn on your phone's flashlight and bring it with you into the bathroom, but place it out of reach.
- Install a night-light.

For more ideas, see the upcoming section Lighting.

When You Have to Use a Mirror

When you're getting ready, or grooming, this is not an exception, not permission to hang out in front of a mirror unprotected. **Apply protectors in these situations too.** For example:

- Wear a face mask, bandana, or both when grooming in front of the mirror, leaving only the area you're grooming exposed.
- Cover blemishes with bandages *before* grooming, trying out hairstyles, or analyzing a certain feature (and don't analyze yourself more than absolutely necessary—e.g., obsess less over what you look like; appreciate the good and forget the rest, or work on it if you can, with a committed and compassionate attitude).

Pass on grooming when stressed, but beware that stressful days might be when you're most drawn to the mirror.

Picking is the way you're used to expressing your stress or relaxing, but it is not the way that leaves you actually feeling good. Build new, healthier, protective habits instead.

- Wait till someone you trust, who can keep you in check, is around.

- Set a timer with an embarrassing alarm and place it halfway across the house (this works great if you have roommates or neighbors).
- To see the movement of your body for exercises, posture practice, or dancing, record yourself and play it back, instead of standing in front of the mirror. Or stand far back from the mirror for these activities.
- Put makeup on with a hand-held mirror to prevent yourself from having a free hand with which to pick or pull. (This doesn't work for me, but it works wonders for others.)
- Keep your hand consciously on the light switch the entire time you're checking yourself out (ideally just a few seconds). If you can't reach your light switch, hold or touch something else, such as the sink nob; you're not allowed to let go of it as you look at yourself. And again, don't look more than necessary.

These *foundational habits* will be helpful as you progress, but as you start following the steps outlined here, **consider putting off *all* grooming that may trigger you,** for example, doing your brows or shaving.

In my desire to be diligent so I could finally overcome my dermatillomania, I did this, and the wonderful progress I had right away was so encouraging that it pushed me forward into more healing.

◆

Regardless of what protector you apply, at the first thought of picking or pulling, *leave the mirror.* This is important enough to repeat. When doing mirror activities, at the first thought of your BFRB . . .

Leave the mirror.

Just . . . Stay Away from Mirrors

Unless you have a *good* reason to look in the mirror, like getting ready, just don't look. Don't wander toward the mirror just because, or because you're bored, have nothing to do, or just feel like it.

Or to inspect a cold sore, canker sore, tiny cut, stye, or anything you've already looked at and, honestly, can't do anything about.

Sometimes we do this, and it goes OK. But how often does it not go well? Trust me, this isn't a gamble you want to partake in.

Avoid the mirror at all costs.

◆

When not needing to use the mirror, if you find yourself inches away from it for no good reason, as soon as you realize what you're doing, jut your hand out and push till your elbow is straight so that you back away *that far*. This is certainly an in-the-moment response, a *responsive habit*.

Lighting

Below are ways to manage the lighting, be it in your bathroom, bedroom, living room, or anywhere else you visually search for BFRB targets.

Remove Excess Bulbs

Remove a few lightbulbs if your lighting is needlessly bright due to an abundance of bulbs. If that's not possible, maybe using lower-wattage bulbs is.

Install a Night-Light

Night-lights are an extremely convenient protector, one I use myself in the bathroom and bedroom.

- Motion-activated night-lights pop on before you reach for the light switch.
- A push-light or an LED dimmer-switch can be placed next to the switch to train you to go for that instead of the regular light.
- Inexpensive, plug-in night-lights can be plugged in once evening hits.

Consider stashing a night-light in your bag or purse when you visit family or go on trips. This way, you can control your new environment.

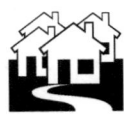

New environments (hotel rooms, friends' bathrooms, public restrooms) might lull you into making exceptions, but continue to stay far from the mirror, keep lighting dim, avert your eyes from targets, and practice all your other protectors.

Try Colorful Bulbs

Bulbs that are just like regular ones except that they're red, green, blue, orange, etc., can be found online. Colorful bulbs make it hard to see details on the skin but still provide sufficient light. (If you can only find "smart" bulbs, set the color that suits you, and hide the remote, so you can't easily make the light bright again in order to pick.)

Possibly not practical in the bathroom or other common areas (depending on who you are and who you live with), these colorful bulbs can be great for bedrooms (I use them in mine).

"Smart" lights, which can be programmed to change color or dim at certain times of day, are also great (again, hide the remote once you've set the lights).

If need be, talk to those you live with. But take matters into your own hands. Don't ask for the lighting or mirror placements to be changed; ask if they mind, and then do it yourself so you can guarantee it happens right away.

Use Glasses

Glasses can be an aid. For example:

- Take off prescription glasses before going into the bathroom.
- Wear blue-light-blocking glasses at night.
- Keep sunglasses on when entering public bathrooms.

Be Candlelit

Use the bathroom and shower/bathe by candlelight. This is not only protective but also pleasant!

Bathing and Showering

Below are more ways to protect while bathing, showering, and just being in the bathroom.

- Keep *every single* potential picking tool (e.g., tweezers, bobby pins) out of the bathroom when you're not using them for (protected) grooming.
- Decide when the least triggering time to bathe or shower is (e.g., morning or evening?).
- To avoid feeling bumps, wash your body with a loofah (especially if you have a triggering blemish or breakout somewhere on your body).
- To avoid feeling bumps, wash your face with a clean rag or facial sponge (especially if you have a triggering blemish or breakout on your face), or splash water up to it without touching it.
- Avert your eyes from triggering areas while bathing.
- Do not hang out around mirrors before or after showering. Get in and out.

Some turn on the water as soon as they enter the bathroom. The wasting of water and the persistent rushing sound is a cue to get in there asap.

- Learn where the best place to dress/undress is. What place is the dimmest, the least tempting? Bathroom or bedroom?
- Have your clothes picked out *before* showering, to avoid too much time with exposed skin.

◆

Over time, these *foundational* and *responsive* habits and *barriers* to do with mirrors, lighting, and triggering locations should become the way of life. In return, you'll have the clearer skin, fuller hair, or longer lashes you seek.

Products and Personal Care

If time spent on skin, hair, or nails seems trivial, again think about how much time you spend picking, pulling, or biting. The right products and personal care habits allow you to focus in a *helpful* way on these areas you tend to, for lack of a better word, obsess over.

I highly recommend creating beauty and personal care routines. Knowing that they're good for your healing, you may actively appreciate these routines too, as a way to foster joy and relax.

◆

Even if you don't target blemishes, you may find this first section—Skin Care—helpful.

If you have preferences or doctor-ordered guidelines that negate any of the below, disregard it.

Skin Care

I can't overstate the importance of skin care—or anything that allows you to prevent whatever you target, and there are lots of things to target on the skin.

Take blemishes.

When you consider that a factor behind blemishes is dead skin becoming trapped in your pores, you see how important exfoliation, which removes dead skin cells, is. So, let's start there.

Exfoliation

Alpha and beta hydroxy acids (AHA and BHA) are popular, effective exfoliants, which help with:

- Shallow scarring
- Active breakouts
- Preventing pimples
- Post-inflammatory marks (discoloration)
- Wrinkles

I buy a lot of my skin care, including exfoliants, from Paula's Choice because the brand is effective, not tested on animals, and free of fragrances. It's somewhat expensive, but the products are top quality, and they last a long time. Timeless Skin Care is another brand I buy. (Maybe you already have brands you trust. Check those for acids.)

> *With AHA, you will be more sun-sensitive, so please wear sunscreen, use your AHA only on places that'll be covered with clothing (e.g., legs), or stick to BHA.*

◆

A bonus with acids (as well as enzymes—and any other "chemical exfoliant") is that you put them on and walk away. This means less time in front of the mirror or looking at your skin and thus less chance of becoming sucked into a session.

Scrubs, brushes, dermaplaning, and other "mechanical exfoliants" *can* be useful in addition to, or instead of, chemical exfoliants, but if you incorporate them, remember the mirror and lighting protectors from earlier.

And be gentle.

Don't scrub too hard or exfoliate too often, as over-exfoliating can be harmful.[5] While chemical exfoliants can be used once to twice a week, or daily, mechanical exfoliation should probably be done no more than weekly, depending on your skin.

◆

If you don't exfoliate consistently yet, start experimenting till you have a routine that works for you, especially if you pick at blemishes, ingrowns, or other bumps.

Set a reminder to exfoliate if you need to.

Tretinoin

Often discussed in the world of skin care, tretinoin, which is a vitamin A derivative, is technically a medication. It helps with:

- Rebuilding collagen
- Shallow scarring
- Active breakouts and acne
- Preventing pimples
- Post-inflammatory marks (discoloration)
- Wrinkles

No product will undo all the effects of chronic skin picking, or get rid of blemishes completely (your diet and more play in), but thankfully, *many* can help, and in my experience, tretinoin is at the top of the list.

Though some see changes right away, for most the benefits aren't visible for weeks or months, so tretinoin requires consistency over many months. Some people even keep up with it their whole lives (for anti-aging), though it's important to protect from the sun while using it (so, night-time use is best, and wear adequate sunscreen every day).

If you're interested in the wrinkle-reducing, collagen-building, scar-improving effects of tretinoin, inform yourself: watch videos, read articles, and talk to a professional, especially if you take other medications, are a teen, or have health conditions.

Tretinoin brand names include Retin-A and Stevia-A. Dermatologists can prescribe it (though you can ask your primary care doctor if they will). I buy mine from ReliableRxPharmacy.com. If you're an adult, and you don't have health insurance and/or are on a tight budget, this may be a great option for you.

If you have sensitive skin, you can integrate over-the-counter **retinol** (which is also a *retinoid* but is not as strong) into your routine instead.

Sunscreen

Sunscreen can help or hurt your BFRB.

It prevents post-inflammatory marks (that discoloration that can appear after you pick) from getting worse, and preserves **collagen and elastin**.[6] That said, for some, certain sunscreens can cause blemishes.

However, for its usefulness in protecting the skin from picking consequences and aging, and for being a companion to the previous products mentioned, the sunscreen search is well worth it.

Here are some basics to consider:

- Notice whether your sunscreen clogs your pores. If you suspect it does, try a different one and see what happens.

  By bringing pimples to the surface of the skin faster, some products cause "purging," making skin look worse before it gets better. Others, like some sunscreens, just cause breakouts.

- The next issue is a white cast. If you don't detect a white cast in person, see if one appears in photos that use flash. Chemical sunscreens don't leave that chalkiness, but they may not be as effective as physical sunscreens (depending on the ingredients). Thankfully, certain physical sunscreens leave less of that chalkiness, or contain a tint that counteracts it.

  Sunscreens can be "chemical" or "physical."

- Go for a **broad-spectrum** sunscreen (aka, one that protects against *both* UVA and UVB) with **SPF 30** or higher.
- Apply the sunscreen to your face, neck, chest, ears, hands, arms—anywhere your skin will be exposed. The

recommendation is to do this daily, even indoors due to brightness from windows. Although on days the UV index is two or below, it's OK to skip it.[7] Check your weather app.

- Wear enough sunscreen—several pumps, so you can cover your skin in an even layer.

◆

The sun is healthy! Getting sun during the day can help us sleep better at night,[8] among so many other benefits, but opt to get sun *before* 10:00 am or *after* 4:00 pm if you're going to bask unprotected.

Also, not to worry—the sun is reaching you despite your sunscreen, through a bit of unprotected skin here and there, as well as through your clothes.

Miscellaneous

For basics like face wash, toner, and moisturizer, I look for simple, gentle products. I also mind my laundry detergent, conditioner, and more.

To help prevent breakouts, depending on how sensitive your skin is, fragrance-free laundry detergent for pillow cases, towels, and clothes is a good idea, as is washing these items regularly—e.g., weekly or after one use—depending on what the item is.

Additionally, your creamy hair conditioner may be contributing to breakouts, so rinse the conditioner out *before* soaping up.

> Think about what comes in contact with your skin, be it skin care, hair care, or something else. Can you make a change to prevent blemishes or irritation that may cause you to pick?

◆

For the most successful skin care habits, a little research is in order.

For example, I had no idea the tiny, skin-colored bumps around my knees were called "keratosis pilaris" and that they could be smoothed out by using a lactic acid lotion daily. Now my knees are smoother than ever. If you have these bumps on your legs or arms, try this (but you have to be *consistent* over weeks to months).

You too may have skin conditions that are unknown to you. While non-BFRBers may see them as unimportant, for us the mystery bumps, pores, and patches can be part of the vicious cycle of scabs and sores.

To start your research, subscribe to a few trusted skin care channels on YouTube, like the ones listed in the resources at the end of this guide.

✦

Aside from being a *foundational habit*, skin care can be a *responsive habit*: Suppose you're headed to the bathroom to pick—you want to turn back, but you have too much momentum.

Decide that once you get there, you'll instead wipe the blemish with witch hazel, wash your face, shower, or do something *else*.

This may not always work—the momentum toward picking may be too big—but as you keep following these steps and gain confidence and momentum in your healing, you'll be able to stick to that decision more and more.

✦

Even if you don't target your hair or scalp, you may find some useful tips below.

Hair and Scalp Care

Modify your hair care so it includes protective *foundational habits*. For example:

- Wash your hair more often if greasy strands are a trigger.
- At a time you usually pick or pull, rub oils meant to stimulate hair growth into your scalp, e.g., rosemary oil,[9] as a way to soothe yourself instead, and to help regrowth (be sure to dilute essential oils with a carrier like castor or coconut oil).

To avoid oil build-up, which can lead to dandruff,[10] *incorporate a clarifying shampoo once a week or so. If you've never tried a clarifying shampoo, you may be surprised at the difference it makes.*

- If itchiness is a trigger, get to the bottom of your itchy scalp Exfoliation, moisture, and more or less protein[11] in your hair care can help.

Hair care can also be a *responsive habit*. Instead of picking or pulling, you can do the above, or:

- Wet your hair, so you're less tempted to pick at your scalp or pull out strands now that the textures are different.
- Dunk your head in a sink or bowl full of ice water to calm sensations (yes, some BFRBers do this, and not only does it work, it's worth it to them).

These aren't exactly hair care, but they help your BFRB!

Use these ideas to find protectors that may work even better for you.

◆

Even if you don't target your hands or feet, you may find the following helpful. Tips for other BFRBers are sprinkled throughout.

Cuticle, Nail, Hand, and Foot Care

Frayed nails or dry, flaking skin around the nails is a trigger for those who focus on fingers. To protect, incorporate products and do chores differently. For example:

- After you shower, moisturize your toes, heels, and fingers (or any part of you that gets rough, dry, and pickable). **Do this most of the time, if not every time.**
- Wear dish gloves while doing dishes (to prevent drying out the skin and making it more pickable).
- Avoid extra-hot water when hand-washing.
- In the winter, wear gloves outside to protect the skin.
- Carry moisturizer with you (in your coat, backpack, purse,

etc.). At home, have various moisturizers in useful spots (near the sink, next to the bed).

For moisturizing, consider:

- **Lotions and balms**—Not all feel greasy (a complaint some have), and some are more moisturizing than others.
- **Vaseline or Aquaphor**—It's amazing what this will do to the skin around the nails when applied regularly.
- **Cuticle oils**—I enjoy the brand Delore Nails. This product is also a nail hardener—which may help those who compulsively peel their nails.

It can take trial and error to find the thing that will offer you the most benefit, so buy small bottles to try things out, and get started!

◆

Along with the *foundational habits* above, try these *responsive habits*:

- So you're not tempted later, clip or file nails and hangnails now (new mantra: *clip, don't pick*). Keep nail clippers, or a file, on you.

  If you also pick at blemishes, clippers without the file attachment will be best (otherwise you might use the file to dig out blemishes). Soon, you'll learn what works for you and what triggers you. Adjust accordingly.

- When you have an urge to engage in your BFRB, or even once you've caught yourself engaging in it but are still near the edge and can backtrack, slather moisturizer on your hands *instead*; this is a **go-to action**. Keep moisturizer near locations in which you pick (desk, bed, couch).

  BFRBers with all types of behaviors can try this moisturizing trick, as it offers something else to do.

Manicures

Not wanting to take away from a fresh manicure, many finger pickers abstain from making the skin on their fingers red and raw after a manicure.

You may like the idea of a gel manicure on your natural nails or of getting artificial nails.

Artificial Nails

Combined with other protectors and your increased awareness, the acrylics you tried before or never thought would make a difference in your BFRB can actually help now, though if you're not into fake nails, disregard this and focus on the myriad other protectors. However, I know of one BFRBer who decided to *become* a fake nails person, because of how much it helped her finger picking when she tried it.

As for blemish pickers and others, while it's still possible to pick with fake nails, it's more difficult, offering a bit of a *barrier*.

Though salons are an option, pharmacies and box stores sell sturdy press-ons nowadays, and you can find hacks online for how to make them last even longer, if you want.

Pedicures

Getting regular pedicures may help if rough skin on your feet is a trigger, though you can also do things on your own. For exfoliation (once skin is healed), I'm a big fan of the Mr. Pumice Extra-Coarse Pumi Bar.

Remember to moisturize your feet after showering too.

◆

Even if you don't target your lips, you may find Lip Care helpful.

Lip Care

Because dry, pickable lips are a trigger for pickers, lip care is a huge protector. It includes:

- Don't lick your lips; this only dries them out further after the moment of temporary relief[12] (and may have you feeling pickable things with your tongue).
- Keep a water bottle nearby so you drink plenty of water (from my own experience and that of others, more hydration taken internally results in less chapped, plumper-looking lips).
- Use lip balm often. Keep various balms in designated places, such as your desk, nightstand, car, jacket, backpack, and purse. Vaseline and Aquaphor can work too.

Not only will regularly using lip balm keep pickable things at bay (*foundational habit*), but you can apply it when you have the urge to pick, in the moment (*responsive habit*). That is, when you get an urge, or right after diverting from your BFRB, apply lip balm, as a different response. This is also a **go-to action**.

◆

Other ways to help with lip picking and biting:

- Use a lip scrub once or twice a week to slough off dry, dead skin (don't go too hard and don't do this too often). Buy one or make your own, e.g., sugar and honey.
- Try numbing gloss or balm; some also enjoy the stimulating tingle.
- Find your lipstick shade and make it your signature color, i.e., wear it often. The idea is that not wanting to smear your lipstick in public (or at home) will help you abstain from picking.

◆

Regardless of your BFRB, if shave bumps and ingrown hairs are a problem, read on for smooth-shave tips.

Shave Better to Reduce Bumps

Despite attempting to address my ingrown hair problem throughout my life, ultimately I was cheap and I didn't want to litter the planet with old razors, so I kept dull razors for weeks and lathered with soap. As I began healing my dermatillomania and realized the bumps were a big trigger, shaving better fell into place.

Ingrowns are hard to get rid of entirely, but for fewer bumps (and thus fewer sessions), I recommend the following—it applies to legs, underarms, beards, and more.

1

Use a Sharp Razor

Switch out your blade every three shaves or so. Razors can be expensive, but safety razors are a workaround. You can buy a box of blades for less than the cost of a conventional razor. The metal base of a safety razor is refillable, and the metal blades are recyclable (put them in a metal can before tossing them in the recycling bin).

It can take practice to use this style of razor, but those who've made the switch with me find that it's worth it.

2

Exfoliate Shave Areas

Do this every time *before* shaving (e.g., apply a BHA), or do it regularly throughout the week as part of your skin care routine.

3

Use Shaving Cream

Eos Shaving Cream and Nicel Bioactives Shave in the Shower Gel are products I enjoy (they're non-drying and non-irritating), though a gentle hair conditioner will do the trick.

◆

If a smoother, cheaper, more environmental shave sounds good to you, put a safety razor and blades in your to-buy list, along with shaving cream and exfoliants.

Even doing one of the things above, or upping your shaving in some other way, will help. And if you have the means, laser hair removal is a fantastic idea.

A final tip: if within a few days your fresh shave becomes a breakout zone—shave down instead.

Straighten Your Posture

Straightening up offers a jolt of well-being and confidence. While negative emotions are triggers, positive emotions keep picking, pulling, and biting at bay. Straightening up *may* look like:

- Relax the back of the neck completely.
- Open up the chest.
- Bring the shoulders down and back.
- *If standing*, tuck your tailbone (or pelvic bone) in to the degree that you have a slight, natural bend in the knees.
- Keep feet about shoulder-width apart and pointing forward, with your weight distributed evenly between them.

A shortcut is to aim your solar plexus at the sky and relax as much as possible.

This can take practice! And of course we all have different bodies, so this may be different for you.

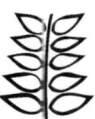

I hold my ideal posture as long as I can to help retrain my muscle memory, since I'd like good posture to come effortlessly to me. If I can't maintain it for even a few seconds, this may mean I'm exhausted or worn out and need to rest as soon as I can.

A different posture indication that applies to many of us: leaning forward in one's seat or while walking can be a sign of not living in the present, of being anxious about whatever is *next, next, next.*

Lean back. Settle into now. Slow down.

Perking up when you notice you're slouching will have cumulative effects. As your posture stays steady over time, you'll only feel better, helping to keep triggers at bay. However, in response to intense emotion, some sit up straight and take several deep breaths.

As you can see, straightening up can be a *foundational habit* and a *responsive habit.*

Recruit Family and Partners

Family members have probably scolded you or advised you to "just stop" in a misguided attempt to help. But even if they don't understand the drive, once they know it's a disorder and that you're committed to stopping, they can be a surprisingly effective protector.

Recruit trusted people to ask/tell you to stop if they catch you engaging in your BFRB, or if they see you're about to. Let them know that now that you're more informed about BFRBs and healing in earnest, you'll do your best to listen.

If you don't find it helpful to be told to stop (it annoyed me before these steps, but I'm incredibly grateful now), ask someone you trust to *point out* when you're picking or pulling, or angling to. Ask them to alert you via gentle touch, a certain word, a question (e.g., "Hey, did you realize you're picking?"), or some other cue.

If you use grooming tools for your behavior (e.g., tweezers, brow razors), have someone hide these for you until you need them for grooming *and nothing else.*

◆

As you progress, having conversations about what is or isn't working (for you and them) is natural, and helpful.

Speak Up

You know when you realize what you're doing, but even though you want to stop, you can't? When you're here, be it at the edge of a session or in the grips of one, muster your voice.

For example:

"Stop"

At the edge of a session, try saying, "Stop," *out loud.*

> *Speaking can snap us out of that trance when we feel it setting in.*

"1 . . . 2 . . . 3"

Counting out loud to three can help you back away from the mirror, or anytime you realize you're scrutinizing and falling into a trance.

Call Out to Someone

My partner, who knows all about my dermatillomania, might hear me say, "Hey, can you come here for a sec?" or "Hey, can you help me?" or "Can you call me over to you?"

> *When I started these steps, while picking, or at the edge, I literally couldn't speak, even when I wanted to. After following them for a bit, I could use my voice as a protector, and I do to this day.*

When one line of defense has been bulldozed, another protector can come into play. Stared for too long, and got too close? Use your voice. Even better, though, is to practice other protectors, particularly those foundational habits, consistently and proactively so you don't find yourself so close to the cliff at all.

Snap or Clap

Using your voice can snap you out of it, but anything that accomplishes this, such as literally snapping, will too. Do this just as you realize you've been picking or pulling, or that you're about to, as a **go-to action**.

Edge Away

What I'm about to say may be obvious, but I wanted to shine a light on it so that if you do it, you know you're on the right track, and so that you can harness it if you don't:

When already engaging in a precursor, we can't always rip ourselves away, but we can sometimes *edge away*. Try this when your head is telling you to stop but your body isn't listening.

For example, in the bathroom, even if your eyes are glued to your reflection or skin, you may be able to maneuver your hands toward the light switch and flick it off. Your eyes will suddenly find themselves in the dark, helping to snap you out of it.

It's like being an octopus, as if your different parts have brains of their own—use this to your advantage.

> *Of course, if your BFRB doesn't involve your hands, you'll edge away differently.*

Immediately after edging away, practice some **go-to action**, like adhi mudra, taking a deep breath, moisturizing, snapping, or grabbing a crystal or another hand-held protector.

◆

> *Feel free to skip upcoming sections on clothing, hair, or gloves, that don't apply to you, if any. Either way, tune in again at Make Yourself Up Daily.*

Protective Clothing

Wearing protective clothing at home has greatly improved the look of my skin. My main piece of advice is to choose clothing *you truly enjoy*—something comfortable—so you'll stick with it.

Ideas include:

Hot Weather

- T-shirts (instead of tank tops)

If you pick your shoulders or chest.

- Capris (the stretchy, breathable ones meant for working out)
- Long skirts
- Long dresses

If you pick your legs.

- Thin, low socks

If you pick your feet.

Cold Weather

- Turtlenecks

- Sweaters

Who doesn't love a cozy sweater? Embrace this as a protector.

- Wrist warmers
- Long sleeves
- Tight-fitting pants

Snug/tight pants and sleeves that you can't easily pull up may be extra helpful in the beginning of your healing. E.g., choose work-out pants over baggy pajama pants.

- Tall socks

Night-Time

Be sure to wear protective outfits at least until the lights are *off*.

From there, if you sleep naked (or nearly), consider keeping a robe near your bed and slipping that on when you have to use the bathroom in the middle of the night.

If you pick in your sleep, try getting used to wearing comfortable protective clothing *to* bed. Consider tight, but breathable, long-sleeve shirts and pants. You may have tried this before with little success, but combined with other protectors discussed (such as de-stressing regularly), it may just help now.

General Clothing Tips

- **Tailor clothing to current targets.** For example, if my chest is clear, I may wear a T-shirt with a low neck. If I have a breakout, I'll opt for a high crew neck so I don't scrutinize my breakout.

- **Change into something more protective right away** if you *try* to wear something less protective one day and it's not cutting it.
- **Cover up any triggering spots**, and double down on other protectors, if you must wear something like a tank top or shorts because it's so hot.
- **Change back into protective clothing** as soon as you return home if you wore a tank top, shorts, or a short skirt out.

Hair and Head Protectors

While you may have tried wraps or wigs before, combined with your growing awareness and a range of other protectors, this can be even more effective now.

If you have trich, or pick at your scalp, consider the following *barriers*:

- Scarf
- Head wrap
- Hat
- Bandana or headband
- A certain hairstyle
- A wig (a fun one or one that mimics your real hair)

You might wear the above at home only, or at work or school too.

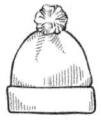

If you pull in your sleep, cover up before bed with a:

- Bonnet
- Scarf
- Microfiber hair towel
- Wig cap

These can also be worn while you're hanging out at home during the day or evening.

◆

Experiment and, to increase the chance you'll stick with head protectors, try things *you truly enjoy* or at least find reasonable.

Gloves

Wearing gloves is effective, and especially at first, it's a protector some might want to rely on. I know of one BFRBer who praises wearing thin gloves at home. After some trial and error, he found the right brand to make this protector reasonable for him.

Others wear light, cotton, dermatological gloves, or even disposable plastic gloves.

If you do your behavior while sleeping, wearing a pair of gloves at night is one idea. You may wriggle them off at first, but with some modification, this can stick.

If not, that's OK.

One protector will not make or break your healing. Try applying bandages, or some of the other protectors mentioned, on your fingertips or on spots before bed instead.

Make Yourself Up Daily

BFRBs can at times be fueled by concern over our looks.

To counter this, consider getting dressed up every single day, even if staying in. Doing this builds confidence and self-appreciation (and this goes for everyone, even non-BFRBers).

Sure, appreciating ourselves in any state is the goal, but taking the time to make yourself up says, *I value you*. It makes you feel like you've got your life together. When you walk by the mirror, even if you look for only a moment, you get to think, *Wow, I look good,* rather than saving that for the rest of the world.

This has made a huge difference in my life as a whole.

As someone who often works from home, I'd hang out in comfy but ugly clothes, my hair a mess. I'd only wear clothes I liked when going out.

Now, while I choose clothes that are on the comfier side, I wear outfits I actually like. I don't put on make-up, but I curl my lashes, smooth out my hair, and choose jewelry that makes me feel powerful.

For you, this will of course look different (maybe you want to wear makeup at home, like lipstick, or you don't get much out of jewelry).

When I'm in an outfit I feel like me in, I take a picture with my phone so I can remember it (a quick picture that doesn't have to look good because it's for my eyes only).

If you like this idea, take a moment right now to create one or all of the following albums:

- **Outfits** (outfits to wear out; they may show target areas)
- **At-Home Outfits** (comfy but nice-looking outfits that cover target areas)
- **Hairstyles**

This habit has been revolutionary in removing that "what to wear?" stress and making me look and thus feel great more often.

Over the Counter

Pain, Tingling, Itching

If you feel pain, tingling, itching, or some other sensation at the moment of an urge:

- Apply a cold pack to the spot or zone.
- Wrap ice in a rag and put it over the spot or zone.

- Apply an anesthetic (i.e., numbing) ointment to the spot or zone.

Please don't ignore a potential medical concern. If you have extreme pain or other signs of a serious infection, or you have any doubt at all over a spot, seek medical attention.

- Place a cold spoon on skin or lashes to numb them. Keep spoons in your freezer so you can grab one when you need it.
- Hair can tickle our faces, prompting us to scratch and then keep scanning for texture. Tie hair back or pin it, or scratch without using your hands (e.g., use a sleeve or a pen).
- Slap or tap an itchy spot, instead of scratching.

Itching is a normal sign of skin healing. If you feel it, try to reframe it as a good thing—it means you're healing!

Hydrocolloid Bandages and Acne Patches

If you haven't tried hydrocolloid bandages, aka blister bandages or "acne patches," they may just become a favorite for you as they are for so many. These bandages draw the gunk from a blemish, so they're *doing something to resolve* that thing you want off your body, in addition to acting as a barrier.

Not just for blemishes, they can go anywhere you have a wound, e.g., heels, fingers, chest, or legs, to speed up healing. As a bonus, hydrocolloid bandages can stay on for a few days.

> Have other protectors in place, such as dim lighting, as you apply these bandages.

To make your supply last, trim large bandages as needed.

◆

Apply over-the-counter protectors regularly as soon as you notice a spot, as a *foundational habit*. They can be a new *responsive habit* too: Suppose some trigger has propelled you toward the bathroom—on the way there, decide you'll instead cover the spot with a bandage once you arrive.

Supplements

There's no switch, and definitely no magic pill, but supplements help some BFRBers. These include:

- **N-acetyl cysteine (NAC)**[13] (helps build glutathione,[14] an antioxidant)
- **Vitamin D**[15] (especially if vitamin D deficiencies are present)
- **CBD oil**[16] (especially if anxiety is a trigger)

See the sources and resources at the end for more information.

If you're curious to try supplements, consider these guidelines and suggestions:

- Choose a **brand** that limits additives, coloring, or fillers—read the label and do a little research.
- Decide on your **dose**—e.g., for NAC, 600 mg twice a day for a **total of 1,200 mg** may be a good place to start, though some up this quantity to around 3,000 mg if they see no results after a few months of consistent use. (Note that stomach pain and other gastrointestinal issues can be a side effect at higher doses—which is one reason to ease in.)
- Determine whether an **additional supplement** will aid your chosen supplement—e.g., some recommend supplementing with vitamin C if using NAC to prevent possible kidney stones. (I couldn't find a study supporting this, but I saw it enough that I'd feel remiss if I didn't mention it.)
- Think on whether you have conditions or take **medications** that might contraindicate the supplement (if you have any doubt whatsoever, talk to a doctor).

- Be patient. It can take **consistent**, committed use over weeks to months before you notice a difference.

While research into BFRBs is increasing,[17] much of the information regarding supplements and BFRBs is anecdotal as of this writing. With a few exceptions (NAC, Vitamin D), recommended supplements for BFRBs focus on triggering mental health conditions, such as anxiety, rather than on the BFRB itself; however, that's promising—as these are related.

◆

Supplements can help. However, identifying triggers and protecting will *still* be necessary if you want to heal. As I said, there's no magic pill.

If you're unsure about supplements, focus on all the other protectors that are readily at hand, and maybe come back to supplements later on.

Balance Your Hormones

Hormones come into play with BFRBs because:

- Urges can heighten around hormonal shifts, which can happen due to puberty, pregnancy, menopause, periods (see next section), and more.
- In some, acne can be linked to a hormonal imbalance (and acne equals picking).

Eating right, sleeping enough, and minimizing stress help balance hormones.[18] However, if you suspect your hormones are off, and you're concerned, you can get your hormone levels checked with a healthcare professional and discuss next steps with them.

Looking up recommendations and tips from others who are experiencing the same things you are (e.g., perimenopause, menopause) may be greatly helpful.

Period Care

Because we may attempt to escape period pain, or the pain can become an added stressor on top of other things we want to escape, periods can be triggering.

Here are a few strategies if you suspect, or know, that urges heighten around your period:

Track It

Download a period-tracking app to help you prepare for your period, e.g., by lessening your work or family load if possible during this time that your energy may be lower (this will help reduce stress and thus the desire to flee by picking).

Drink Teas

Drink raspberry leaf tea for several days *before* as well as during your period. If you experience cramps, you may be as surprised as I was to find that drinking this tea *actually* helps. (We want raspberry *leaf* tea, by the way, not just raspberry tea.)

Cinnamon, ginger, and other teas may also help with cramps.

Bring Warmth

A heating pad or a warm compress can alleviate discomfort. (As a bonus, this natural way avoids pain meds.)

Cut Caffeine

Limit caffeine (or downgrade your source, e.g., switch from coffee to caffeinated tea for the week) if you notice, as many do, that caffeine worsens cramps, a lot.

Expect Bumps

If you break out around your period, first, acknowledge that breakouts right now are normal and, second, prepare to practice all the protectors you've got in your arsenal till hormonal breakouts clear (e.g., bandages, protective clothing, decompressing, etc.).

Reduce Toxicity

Irritation on the inside can negatively influence BFRBs. Something that's "toxic" reacts negatively with you or is poisonous to some degree. To help you reduce toxicity in your environment and body:

- **Eat clean** to *avoid* your intake of toxicity, and eat clean to detoxify. This means, limit food dyes and fillers and foods grown with a high amount of pesticides.
- **Learn about the ingredients** in your beauty, home, car, and personal care products and which ones you may want to avoid.
- **Make sure your water is filtered** or otherwise clean.

Because it's a large topic, I only wanted to plant the seed of avoiding toxicity, and I've included a resource at the end.

Mind Your Mindset

A lot can be said on the topic of thoughts, but it doesn't have to be complicated. Put simply:

> Helpful thoughts do not come from
> fear, lack, or skewed thinking.

Instead, they are:

- Encouraging, compassionate, understanding, loving, and forgiving

Even if you can't get to these right away, reaching these states is usually the goal.

- Solution-oriented
- Resilient
- Calm
- Patient
- Non-judgmental
- Curious

Aka, seek information instead of defaulting to fear or reactivity.

- Open to challenges
- Fun, playful

Make things funny; make light. For example, laugh at your hands' persistence.

- Childlike

Again, tap into fun, innocence, playfulness—not the same as being childish.

- "Self-parenting"

Treat yourself in the caring way you would a child, when you need the extra care or when you find yourself being harsh (i.e., would you talk to a child in a harsh way?).

- Far-reaching

Rather than letting immediate satisfaction fuel you, consider future consequences.

- In line with who you want to be or who you are at your best
- Proportionate

Consider whether you're overreacting and whether you can take it in stride instead.

- Perhaps spiritual, trusting, and full of faith
- & so much more

Whether you do it on paper or in your head, adjusting your thoughts may become a conversation with yourself, with questions, complaints, and objections being answered by more positive, realistic, confident, or soothing thoughts.

Suppose you have the following fear-based, knee-jerk thought during some outing or event—in action, using protective, or **counter**, thoughts looks like this:

⚠ TRIGGER
I feel uncomfortable. I want to leave. Everything's awkward! It's clear I shouldn't have come.

🛡 COUNTER THOUGHTS
It's natural for social interactions to be awkward at first, *as people settle in.*

Everyone is a little awkward. *If I look around, I see it's not just me. And those who aren't awkward at all? They're an inspiration.*

On the one hand, if I'm awkward, I'm being authentic. *So what if I seem as insecure as I feel right now? On the other hand, I can try to appear more confident by being less fidgety. I get to decide.*

◆

I'm not here to convince you conflict and negativity don't exist, just to encourage you to look at it—*whatever* it is—in a way so that you have your own back.

Cheerlead for yourself. Soothe yourself. Encourage and guide yourself. Every moment of every day, protective thoughts never have to leave you.

Dissolve the Mania Mind

Let's apply protective thoughts directly to BFRBs. What better way to counter the skewed thinking of the *mania* mind than with thoughts?

Here are some examples:

⚠ TRIGGER

Wondering, *How is my skin healing after that recent session? Let me go check.*

🛡 COUNTER THOUGHT

My skin is doing better than before, that's for sure! If I look, I may pick and make it worse.

⚠ TRIGGER

Is that blemish ready? Let me go look.

🛡 COUNTER THOUGHT

It doesn't matter whether it's ready, because I've decided to never pick. It'll go away better on its own.

⚠ TRIGGER

The desire to look at skin after feeling texture

🛡 COUNTER THOUGHT

I don't have to look. If I look, I'll probably pick.

⚠ TRIGGER

Fear that something won't go away without help

🛡 COUNTER THOUGHTS

I know from past experience this will go away on its own, even if it takes a while. I'd rather it take a while than leave a permanent mark.

I'm curious how long this will take to heal on its own. I want to see how it'll evolve. It'll be an experiment. (Curiosity.)

⚠ TRIGGER

Seeing a blemish (or feeling a hair) and *needing* it to be *gone*

🛡 COUNTER THOUGHT

What is it I want to do so badly here? (Think about how it's just pus, trapped sebum, and skin cells; or just a piece of skin; just a bulb attached to a strand of hair. Focus on the mundane reality of it to help lessen the drive.)

⚠ TRIGGER

Feeling bad about yourself because you have a blemish or spot

🛡 COUNTER THOUGHTS

It's not nasty or bad for this to be there. Spots are normal and human.

It's OK for this to be here. It can stay.

⚠ TRIGGER

I think this one is ready!

🛡 COUNTER THOUGHT

How many times have I thought that, and it wasn't? Plus, I've decided to never pick.

⚠ TRIGGER

I have to pick this.

🛡 COUNTER THOUGHT

Picking is a choice. (And I choose not to.)

⚠ TRIGGER

I want to pick this.

🛡 COUNTER THOUGHTS

Will I be happy later if I do? (Future-focused, rather than impulsive.)

How will I feel about myself after?

Play out the full scenario.

Picking doesn't help with the emotion, or physical state. *What am I feeling? What do I need?*

→

To protect from triggering thoughts, keep increasing your awareness (Step 1) so that you notice them. From there, counter these with thoughts that are **a)** realistic as well as **b)** in line with the healing you want.

→

Whether you counter a thought directly related to your behavior, or thoughts that feed stress, anxiety, insecurity, and other unpleasant emotions that make you want to escape into your BFRB, the mind is one of your most powerful protectors.

Don't Give Permission

The following are examples of **permission-giving thoughts**. These willful thoughts are not helpful.

⚠ TRIGGER

I've been doing so well! . . . This little bit is OK.

🛡 COUNTER THOUGHT

This will throw a wrench into my feeling of progress, *and I'll regret backsliding. Plus, if I start, no matter what I tell myself, I can't guarantee I'll be able to stop.*

⚠ TRIGGER

This is so tiny, I don't have to log if I pick.

🛡 COUNTER THOUGHT

Why would I not log this? *This is not an exception, no matter how tiny.*

⚠ TRIGGER

It's just one spot.

🛡 **COUNTER THOUGHT**

If I pick that one spot, I'll probably go on to pick more.

⚠ **TRIGGER**

There's clearly stuff in that blemish, so it'll be easy to get.

🛡 **COUNTER THOUGHT**

So often something looks easy and ready, and then it's not. *I'd rather not take the chance of making a permanent scar there.*

⚠ **TRIGGER**

I already started. I might as well get everything now.

🛡 **COUNTER THOUGHT**

I'll be wiring in my BFRB more deeply *if I continue.*

    These thoughts might flash by quickly, but try to catch and decode these blips. The fact that we can catch these, once we try, is good news. It gives us power to change them.

    Let your *mania* mind speak. Listen to it. Respond. Talk yourself through an urge or a session. Ask yourself questions (e.g., "Can I back away? Do I really want to be doing this?").

Balance Your Thoughts

The *mania* mind aside, skewed thinking creeps into other areas of life and, in a roundabout way, leads right to picking. Here are just a few examples of what psychologists call **cognitive distortions**.

    Be on the lookout for . . .

All-or-Nothing Thinking

"This *moment* is going wrong, so *today* is a bad day."

    "I messed up, so I'm a crappy person."

    Just because something isn't going your way right now doesn't mean you have to give up on the day, or your mood. And all messing up means is that you messed up, in regard to one thing, not that you're a bad person.

You may not be having these thoughts outright ("I'm no good"), but you may be feeling *just* like this, whether or not you've put words to it. Start to put words to your feelings. You may be surprised by what they translate to.

Another example:

A no-chewing streak has made you feel invincible, as if your BFRB troubles were a long-ago dream. But as soon as you chew, you feel like you'll never be rid of it, discounting the better-than-ever-streak you just had.

The word is balance. A real view. Not skewed one way or another.

Mind-Reading Thoughts

An example of this is assuming what people think about you with little to no real proof. For example, "They don't like me," or "They think X, Y, and Z about me."

Underestimating Your Ability to Deal and Cope

This gets in the way of you dealing and coping. As I said much earlier, difficulty avoidance leads to picking or pulling, so **empower and encourage yourself to face things instead**. You *can* do it.

Giving More Weight to What's Unwanted

If two good things happened and one bad happened, we still may give more attention to the bad thing. One example is routinely giving more attention to when someone is unreceptive, not paying attention, or disapproving than to when they've shown you their attention or approval.

Process the bad, but acknowledge the good.

Fortune-Telling Thoughts

This is when you're *sure* about something that you actually don't yet know the outcome of. Let's take this example: *Humanity and our planet are doomed.*

This thought is more responsible and productive as:

Not everything is horrendous. Some things are pure and beautiful. Also, many are coming up with solutions; many haven't given up—I'd like to put my energy toward that. Even if the world does end (which, by the way, it inevitably, eventually will), I want to be someone that cared and tried.

•

Look for exaggerations, sweeping judgments, and additional distortions about yourself, others, or the world around you as you go about your day, and challenge them with your protective counter thoughts.

Create More Helpful Beliefs

Left unchallenged, negative, routine thoughts lead to beliefs that can bring us down unnecessarily. For example:

- *To make a lot of money I have to work a lot more than I want to.*
- *If I have a lot of money, my friends will no longer want me around just for me.*
- *If I have a lot of money, people may see me as stuck up.*

Whether you realize you have these beliefs or not, they can keep you from taking concrete steps to starting a business or forging toward a certain profession, even though these things aren't necessarily true.

See these counter thoughts:

- *Opportunities exist to make money without working my days away. This isn't to say it's easy to find them (though it might be), but it's possible, and this is my goal.*
- *I can decide to simply help those close to me if and when they have a financial need I can help with* (magnanimous thinking)*; I acknowledge there's a difference between being greedy and opportunistic and being in need. I can also set boundaries. If people can't understand my boundaries around money, then possibly they aren't the best people to have around.*
- *If I remain the humble and grounded person that I am, I'll be perceived that way.*

•

Limiting beliefs *will* have you behaving in destructive ways. And others, sensing your subtle cues, will respond to your beliefs. This can affect romantic relationships, friendships, or professional relationships.

Here's another example of a limiting belief:

Finding the type of partner (or friends) I want is difficult.

Your subconscious works to prove it's right, to become right—so you might put yourself in situations that confirm this belief. You may try too hard, thinking that you have to (a turn off). You may not try at all, thinking there's no point (getting you nowhere).

Here's another one:

Getting older says X, Y, and Z about me.

Another way to look at it is that getting older just means you've been here for a while.

At the most basic level, things can be simple and neutral. We give them meaning. So why not give them a meaning that's helpful?

◆

I chose the examples of money, romance, and age because they tend to be relatable, but limiting beliefs can be about anything.

For example, I realized my desire to travel and acquire a lot of knowledge was met with the odd thought that I *didn't want* to be happier, more successful, or living with more ease than others. Because I don't want to leave anyone behind.

However, I can help those around me more, show them what's possible, if I'm at my best. Rewriting this belief was easy—but only when I recognized it was there.

Notice unhelpful beliefs as they come up, or to start living better sooner, set time aside to purposely meditate on limiting beliefs you may have. Ask yourself:

- *Is this true? Or do I just fear that it might be?*
- *Is it really this one way?*
- *Does everyone think like that?*
- *Have I ever seen an exception?*
- *Are my beliefs around this topic helpful?*

Good places to start are beliefs around careers, relationships, family, health goals, achievements you crave, and of course, your BFRB.

Be aware as your *mania* mind twists things that are meant to *help*. A few examples:

⚠ TRIGGER

I do use my BFRB to de-stress, huh? Nothing de-stresses me like this. Nothing is as good.

🛡 COUNTER THOUGHTS

Nothing may be "as good," but it's worth it for me to do whatever I can to stop.

I haven't tried every de-stressing tactic I know.

⚠ TRIGGER

Once I start picking, I can't stop.

🛡 COUNTER THOUGHT

It can be difficult to exit a session, but it's not impossible. *I know because sometimes I can do it.*

◆

As your *mania* mind notices your BFRB going away, it may find ways to make you double down on picking or pulling—it may evolve, get smarter and louder, but its days are numbered now that you're talking back.

Mantras and Affirmations

A *mantra* is a word, sentence, phrase, or question that calls up some wanted state of being. Similar, an *affirmation* encourages the version of your BFRB, your life, or you that you'd like to see (or which you have when you're at your best).

For example, when I quit drinking, a mantra I turned to was:

Wild, tough, and fun naturally. (That is, I don't need alcohol to be these things—I am wild, tough, and fun on my own!)

Another example, one I use when I'm being self-critical or doubtful: *What if I revered everything I did?* or *What if everything I did, I revered?*

The best affirmations are ones whose wording resonates with us (which may change from day to day).

Here are examples you might like to try for yourself. Mantras and affirmations can be applied to all areas of your life, but let's focus on:

Confidence

- *I can handle anything.*
- *I am doing everything right; everything is going right.*
- *I don't have to be perfect; just better than before.*
- *I'm not perfect.* (Takes the pressure off.)
- *You've got this.*

Try both "I" and "you" phrases. "You" reminds us of when someone else praises and validates us,[21] which we can use sometimes.

Self-Love

- *I am inherently worthy.*
- *I approve of myself.*
- *I live in love, not fear.*

Night-Time

- *I will wake up refreshed.*
- *Nearly comfortable and I can sleep. I do not need to be perfectly comfortable.*

BFRB

- *My skin is a miraculous healing organ.*

- *I trust my skin to heal on its own.*
- *My hair grows fast and strong.*
- *Healing is easy.*
- *For me, this process is easy.*

Intentions

Rather than seeing how it'll be and then seeing how you feel after (aka, letting life and others dictate), with intentions you *choose* how it'll go.

For example:

- *I don't want to go to this event, but I'm going to be a good sport.*
- *I'm going to have fun at this outing. I'm going to be fun and easy-going.*
- *I'm going to have a good work day.*

You may be surprised how big of a difference an intentional attitude makes.

◆

Record mantras, affirmations, and intentions somewhere.

> *I keep my personal mantras, affirmations, and intentions in my note app. I also scribble them on scraps of paper I leave around my house, like on my bureau.*

As a *responsive habit,* access them when you need a boost. As a *foundational habit,* review these at regular points in your day or week (or try an app that makes affirmations pop up on your phone).

Listening to affirmations, via YouTube for example, can be foundational or responsive.

Mantras and the like are also fantastic **go-to actions** when used to counter thoughts that are about to throw you over the cliff and into a session. Feel free to take a moment now and create your own BFRB mantra, using everything you've learned so far.

◆

Because of neural pathways, it'll take *repetition*, but sooner than you might expect, you'll find you can shift more easily, and more often, into the best version of you and your life.

Life—*you*—can be fun, serene, sexy, mysterious, successful, adorable, powerful, peaceful, whatever you want, and it starts with your thoughts.

Think the Opposite

What if it were as easy as flipping a negative thought?

Sometimes this is all it takes.

For example, *I'm weak* can be countered by *I'm strong*. An opposing thought like this signals your mind to find evidence for this version of reality, so it will (subconsciously) find the times you've been strong—making you realize you *are* strong.

♦

Though you may feel better instantly, it's also natural to feel discomfort. The trouble with positive thinking is that **if you don't believe it, on any level**, you may actually feel worse after affirming.

If you do, start with a smaller mantra, affirmation, or intention. For example, change *I'm beautiful* to *I have a fantastic smile*. If that's too big, try *I like my smile, I like my teeth*, or *I'm glad I have functioning teeth*.

Find the thought that does make you feel better.

In other words, rather than jumping from really low to really high, climb to your destination, thought by thought. If there's evidence on any level, though, you won't have much trouble with a directly opposing thought.

> *This is where thoughts reach their limit; sometimes we have to create experiences to have as evidence. When we do, we see that great things can happen, that our worst fears don't come true. Even if it's not perfect, or if bad things do happen, we then see we can handle it.*
>
> *For some, the knee-jerk response is to avoid uncomfortable situations, to refrain from risk. But for a more fulfilled life, partake,*

put yourself out there. If you do, discomfort around whatever you want to avoid will lessen. If you keep avoiding things, your aversion and bad feelings toward them can grow.

◆

What negativity do you feel?

Try invoking the complete opposite of it. There's a saying that goes, *the opposite of sick is healed.*

Figuring out the opposite of your current negative feeling or unwanted situation also shows you what you're aiming for. Once you know what that is, aside from affirming it, try the following technique.

Visualization

Picture what you want; what you want people to say to you; what you want to experience. It's OK to let yourself have it. In fact, picturing it can help you let go of limiting beliefs, as it can show you something is more attainable than you might have thought, among other benefits.

When it comes to your BFRB, visualize yourself:

- **With the skin, hair, or nails you want**
- **Being faced with a blemish or hair and not engaging in your BFRB** (think of it as safe rewiring, at a distance)
- **Practicing your protectors** (e.g., see yourself flicking the light off in your bathroom—think of it as additional training and rewiring)
- **As a version of you who doesn't have a BFRB at all** (what do you wear? what do you do in those moments you currently pick? how do you feel? who are you without your BFRB?)

Visualization—your imagination—isn't just wishful. It's a useful tool. The mind deals with, not only words, but with pictures, symbols, and images.[22]

If nothing else, it can make you feel good.

◆

As a *responsive habit,* visualize when faced with triggers or an urge; as a *foundational habit*, work visualization into your life on a regular basis, or visualize whenever you remember to, about your BFRB and beyond.

Act as If

Holding beliefs up to the light to see how they may be limiting you; repeating mantras and affirmations; setting intentions . . . bring these together by *acting as if*.

Maybe work stresses you out, but imagine how much less stressful it'll be if you act as if you are capable, successful, professional. How might you behave? How might you feel? Feel it. Be it.

If you want to be successful at something, how will you feel, act, think, or be once you are? Feel it. Be it.

Act as if you look the way you'd like to, already. Who says you have to wait till you actually do? How might you behave when you do, or if you did? After all, you want to look, or be, that way, so you can *feel like this*.

Take the shortcut.

Others will see you differently. You'll feel happier, your self-esteem will rise, and because of this, you will, in fact, look better, perform better, be closer to your goals.

You have nothing to lose.

Beyond calling up the feelings, acting as if may mean you dress like the person you want to be and you say/do things that are more in line with who that person is. This doesn't mean you take on more than you're prepared for, just that you start to behave more like your ideal.

◆

You are healing, definitely, but because of all the work you've put in and the way you now understand your BFRB, in a way, you're healed already.

However, rather than thinking, *I can stare in the mirror because I'm acting as if I don't have dermatillomania*, this might go like:

Leaving the lights dim/protecting is easy for me because I'm healed.

Healing and healed—take on this dual mindset to put yourself in a better position to succeed.

The alternative is to be the person who's *striving* to change, forevermore.

In other words, don't strive. Be.

To be who you want to be . . . be who you want to be.

And when you forget to—as soon as you remember, inhabit those feelings again, and again, and again. This is rewiring.

Acknowledge and Accept

Because they have overlap, *acknowledge* and *accept* are sometimes used interchangeably, or each is used to mean a slightly different thing.

Both will help you heal.

Acknowledging is recognizing something as real—as valid. Looking at it. **Acceptance**, in one sense, means making peace with the fact that something *is* real. Whether we're OK with it or not, we surrender to the fact that *it's real*.

This *does* mean reaching a level of okayness, but accepting doesn't mean we can't **a)** want to change something, **b)** actively take steps to change it, or **c)** given the option, prefer something didn't happen or wasn't true. Aka, **it doesn't mean we approve of it.**

It just means choosing to no longer be deadlocked with reality. Acceptance stops that struggle that happens within us as we deny, suppress, resist, or ignore something.

It allows relief and peace.

Though I'll bring this right back to BFRBs soon, intrusive thoughts offer a perfect example. Many have intrusive thoughts here and there, but some regularly experience these knee-jerk, extra-unwanted (sometimes taboo and violent) thoughts. My original tactic was to push away my own intrusive thoughts. While understandable, this only caused them to push back, i.e., they'd stay or grow in intensity. This is just how thoughts and emotions work sometimes.

What helped me more than anything was acknowledging and accepting intrusive thoughts as a whole, as well as thought by thought. I calmly repeat, *I acknowledge the thought, and it doesn't bother me. It doesn't bother me. It doesn't bother me* . . . until the thought passes.

Keeping stress low also helps, so if you experience intense intrusive thoughts, that's another reason to de-stress regularly.

> *While I've emphasized the power of thoughts, sometimes a thought is just a thought, not a reflection of who you truly are or*

where you are in life. At the end of the guide, I link a resource on OCD, which can be behind intrusive thoughts.

◆

The previous example aside, the thing we're refusing to accept could be an unwanted medical or mental health condition, part of our identity, a physical attribute, a life circumstance, or an attitude or decision taken by another. Regardless, **by refusing to look at something crappy, we believe we're avoiding pain.** So we may blame others and ignore our part; lie to ourselves; wonder why we're so confused, when it's that we're not *comfortable* enough with the truth to let ourselves recognize it; and so on.

Though sometimes it's not as big as all that.

We just have to train ourselves to look, to let reality in rather than habitually tense against it.

Whether or not you approve of it, or whether you believe others will, accepting the truth—possibly, *your* truth—releases push-back so that you can move forward.

◆

Acknowledging or accepting is often a necessary first step for change or improvement. That said, **acknowledging or accepting is sometimes enough**, the only step needed for immediate ease and progress.

Acknowledge Urges

In line with everything discussed, if you resist, deny, suppress, or ignore an urge, it may stay or grow. So, instead, acknowledge and accept urges. This helps lessen their intensity. For example, you can think:

- *Yes, I want to pick that.* (Acknowledge.)
- *It's OK that I have this urge.* (Accept rather than resent.)
- Call up your *whys* for stopping. (Shift rather than resist.)
- *This hair is different. And that's OK.* (Accept.)
- *Even though I'm working on reducing blemishes and breakouts, when they come, they're OK.* (Accept.)

Accept Your BFRB

What if you never heal your BFRB? Will you simply be unhappy forever?

What if you aim to be OK—happy—even if you have to live with it for the rest of your life, *to accept yourself despite your BFRB?*

Ironically, **this surrendering is part of how many heal.**

By stopping the pointless struggle of wishing you never had to *try* to heal (because it can be tough, or annoying), that you never *had* your BFRB (the regret over the scars and patches), your energy can go in a more useful direction, setting you up for the attitude needed to heal.

In other words, accept your BFRB so you can fully embrace the challenge of healing it.

Accept the Way You Look

Let's suppose you've left permanent marks, or your hair still hasn't grown back in certain areas. The more helpful option is to accept your appearance, every single aspect of it, feel peace with the reality, rather than deny it, fight it, and curse it every step of the way for the rest of your life.

> *A bonus for those triggered by mirrors: accepting what we see in the mirror means less time obsessing in front of it, and thus less picking or pulling.*

How often do you regard yourself, your body, your face, with critiques, desires for improvement, regret?

How often do you regard yourself with love and gratitude?

In another sense, *acceptance* is letting some truth in, making it a part of you, owning it.

> Owning who we are, what we look like, our flaws *and* shining attributes, is a shortcut to confidence.

Break Through the Discomfort

I'm not saying accepting is always easy... When we try to accept, a discomfort may come as we break through a film of resistance and adjust to a new reality. Other times, we're met not with a film but with a wall.

We *refuse* to accept.

Because the relief that comes from it is so worth it, though, here are tips for when acceptance *is* hard (think of something you're having trouble accepting in your life right now and apply the following to it so you can see how it works):

- Think about *any* and all good aspects of this thing.
- Think about any good that came *from* it, or that came to you *despite* it.
- Consider what you *can* do to change or affect it, directly or indirectly, in a way that'll make a big impact or at least offer enough of a shift to make you feel better. Then, put your attention on that.
- Don't *focus* on it (when you can help it). If you really have zero sway or say over something (e.g., on a stranger's opinions), why put your energy there? Focus on what you do like, on what is good, on what you can be grateful for. And hold on to these beautiful things for dear life.

Question Yourself, Know Yourself

All the sections on protective thoughts hinge on whether or not you do this:

Get to the bottom of all issues that bring difficult emotions or discomfort. Maybe it's something you saw, or something someone said. Or something you've been dragging around in your mind for years that comes up from time to time.

As always, journaling is a fantastic tool, and can be done routinely as a *foundational habit* or as needed as a *responsive habit*. Many find they can go deeper when they journal than when they just think things over, but just thinking it over is an option too.

Either way, being honest and vulnerable, and questioning yourself till you reach the truth of how you're feeling and why, is how you can best protect via counter thoughts in the ways described here (e.g., rewriting limiting beliefs, creating helpful mantras, taking on new perspectives).

Useful questions are:

- Why is this bothering me?
- Why am I resisting this?
- What am I afraid of?

In my experience, when the details are stripped away, **fear is at the bottom of most negative emotions**: fear of being rejected or unaccepted, fear that you won't have enough, fear that you'll be alone, on and on.

Whatever you're going through, you can find solace, or thrive, but first you must know what you're afraid of, what you'd like to head toward—what's really going on.

To help you do that . . .

Seek Wisdom

Even if you want to understand or help yourself, you may lack the insight to recognize the root of an issue. Or you can find the root, but you don't know a better perspective.

All through your life, you're gaining your own wisdom and experience, but to take a shortcut, seek out others' wisdom.

Books, friends, family, and the internet are tremendous for this.

When I was first ever heartbroken, I was so desperate to feel better that I downloaded an e-book on the topic. I felt pain still, but with my new understanding of how love and attachment work, it was less. I got through it and went on to have many happy relationships, to handle heartbreak better.

Feelings of unworthiness, being too hard on ourselves, friendships or relationships souring, family dynamics—all these things can contribute to a BFRB session, if they're on our minds as we wander near a mirror or a target. Realistically, we won't know how to handle all these situations.

This is where seeking wisdom comes in.

Sometimes it's as easy as typing a specific problem into a search engine, as a *responsive habit*.

However, regularly soaking in wisdom as a *foundational habit* is a game-changer too. For example, almost on a daily basis as part of my routine, I listen to sources that touch on inspirational or spiritual topics, on human psychology (how people work, how *I* work), and more. This has been fundamental for me to not only stay above water, but thrive.

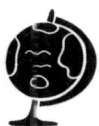

Learning in general—about topics we *actually* enjoy, e.g., space, history, world cultures—reminds us how much exists outside of us, which can be helpful in itself. This is just one way to . . .

Gain Perspective

Specific situations and circumstances require their own wisdom, but gaining some general perspective is helpful too.

For example:

- It could be worse. (Really, it could.)
- What's the worst thing that could happen in this situation?

  Imagining the worst case allows you to prepare for what you'll do if the worst case comes true, which can empower you.

- What can you control about this situation? (Focus on this.) What can you not control? (Let this go as best you can.)
- Do you want to be someone who cares this much about that?

  It's good to care, but sometimes we care too much, about people or topics that may not be the best places to put our limited and precious energy; we may act as if something is the end of the world, focusing too much on one single aspect of the world or some part of our lives.

> By definition, to **stress** is to attach importance to something—to care too much. If you're often stressed, are you caring about a situation too much? Trying to control others' views and behaviors when you can only do so much?

- Is there some other potential explanation, besides the worst-case scenario? (For example, come up with other reasons someone might have done something, like they're having a bad day, or their attention is limited at the moment—any reason other than that something is wrong with you, or something that confirms your fears.)

Grow Over Time

The work of changing beliefs, or feeling better about a subject, is not done all at once. It's OK to shift your focus to relaxation or whatever task is at hand after ruminating on, learning about, or talking about a Big Topic (e.g., identity, a changing relationship, a new stage of your life, where you are in your career).

Some topics are best, or can only be, digested a little at a time. And even then, new topics will emerge; current topics will morph.

> Consider keeping notes on Big Topics. Update these notes as you reach new levels of understanding; jot down conclusions or decisions you've reached. While change may not happen all at once, this can keep you from backsliding.

When we want to immerse ourselves in an experience, go to sleep, or just not think so much, we can bid our thoughts to fizzle out. Especially if we're spinning our wheels on a topic, shifting focus, if for the time being, is best.

Sometimes this is easy.

Other times, our minds devolve into anxious mental chatter. In these moments, tap into techniques discussed earlier, such as adhi mudra, changing your breath, tuning in to the moment, meditation, journaling, and others. Also . . .

Learn to Deal with Heavy Emotion

At times, we can't help but be taken by emotion—we break down. Bringing together some of what we've discussed, and more, here's a list of what to do in those moments when we crack or snap.

Do Not Feed It with Negative Thoughts, Actions, or Words

Just as going down a path of positive thinking has us feeling better and better, traveling down a negative path has us feeling worse and worse. So stay at the precipice of it, be as still as possible, until it passes.

Call Up the New Understanding and Conclusions You've Already Reached

Rather than approaching a topic from a previous level, remind yourself how far you've come with that topic, be it by reading your notes on it, or just thinking it over.

Expel Your Negative Feelings

If need be, express your negative feelings—get them out—as non-destructively as you can. Create art, run, work out, journal furiously, or cry.

Problem-Solve

Rather than giving in to some unwanted reality or feeling defeated by it, be proactive, whether it's by doing something or just by changing your mentality on it.

Think of Positives

Do this unless it results in backlash from yourself. It can be about the issue at hand or about anything else. Things you're grateful for count.

Leave the Room

And if you can't remove yourself from the room, or place, remove your mind from the issue by tuning in to your senses and becoming present.

Accept Imperfection, Marks, Loose Ends, and Uneven Pieces

I'm not talking about your hair, skin, or nails—I'm talking about your life, and the areas within it. Life isn't and will never be perfect. Embrace this about your life, own it.

Don't Become Upset That You're Upset

Negative emotions aren't good or bad, right or wrong; they're natural. So don't beat yourself up for having them. You'll only have more tough emotions on top of the original ones. Also, don't feel angry or resentful that you're experiencing this. Just *experience it*, aka . . .

Feel into It

Many of us feel uncomfortable being in the present moment, just being here, within our bodies. So, to escape, we scan, fiddle, search—pick. But it's not the moment we're escaping from. It's not ourselves, or our bodies. It's whatever discomfort, e.g., fear, anxiety, worry, or pressure, is there.

Feeling into this discomfort helps us to not pick, to not escape. To do this, be still and let whatever feeling is there fill your body.

Follow the sensation.

Enter it.

Observe it.

What's happening in your *stomach*? Your *chest*? Your *throat*? You may feel pressure that you have to breathe through. But you'll find that you can.

> *Emotions have* **physical sensations** *connected to them—whether the sensations are subtle or obvious. These are the sensations I'm focusing on in this section.*

In a way, this acknowledges the discomfort, which, remember, stops that struggle.

Though uncomfortable, an emotion won't kill you. You won't die from feeling this, no matter how bad. (Sometimes we may even resist good feelings, because they can come with a level of discomfort too.)

But as you feel your feelings, or feel *into* them (some also call this "sitting with your feelings"), your feelings transform, and eventually lessen, along with your urges.

Extraction Videos

A protector worth considering is watching extraction videos on YouTube. It's mindless and relaxing, much like actual picking. Note, though, that the people in these videos are *not* doing it themselves—they're getting extractions by experts who've done off-camera pre-work (like disinfecting tools with medical-grade methods, applying professional-grade acids to exfoliate the skin, and more).

That said, not everyone performing extractions in these videos *is* a professional, and sometimes, even if they are, they don't do the best extractions. The videos can still be entertaining, but just remember to not feed your dermatillo-*mania* mind with them.

Because that's a possibility, this protector can be relaxing, or it can be ... triggering.

If you start to feel an urge, watching these types of videos is *not* what you should be doing in that moment. Look at your thoughts. Are you thinking, *This is fun to watch*, or ... *It'd be nice to pick right now. Do I have anything like this on me right now?*

If watching extraction videos leads to a session more often than not, adjust this protector or decide that it just isn't for you, that this isn't something you should do with your time.

> *You'll learn soon enough if well-meaning protectors, like this one, will trigger you rather than help you.*

Bundle Activities

Bundling activities where our hands would otherwise be free to roam protects us. For example:

- Knit or crochet *while* talking on the phone.
- Mend clothes (e.g., socks) *while* watching a show, video, or movie.

- Color *while* watching videos.
- Walk on a treadmill *while* reading.
- Rake the sand in a mini zen garden *while* watching online lessons.

Before bundling, part of us (the mind) is focused, while the remainder (the body) is restless. With bundling, we're fully engaged, mind and body, and thus, we're protected.

To-Do Lists

Disorganization and aimlessness open us up to picking. To-do lists are a great way to counter this.

Here are a few basics:

- **Create your list when it makes the most sense for you**, e.g., the night before; in the morning; and/or throughout the day as items come up.
- **Keep your to-do list realistic.** You'll only have time and energy for a limited number of tasks in a day.
- **Write even small things down**, so they aren't taking up room in your head as you try not to forget them.

You can also have a to-do "dump" for items that fall under "should do at some point, but not urgent."

Easy ways to keep a to-do list are:

- Carry a **physical notebook** in your purse or backpack, or keep it permanently at your desk.
- Download a **to-do list app**.

- Create a note in your **note app** and update it daily.

A to-do dump can go in the back of your agenda, at the bottom of your current to-do note, or in a separate note.

I used to manage my to-do list in a Google Keep note. Now I carry a physical agenda. It's normal for the ways you stay organized to evolve.

Lessen Resistance Around Starting

Sometimes, starting is the hardest part. Overwhelmed by the idea of starting a task, BFRBers may meander into a BFRB session.

Here are some suggestions:

Visualize Yourself Doing It

This will help you feel more comfortable, because you'll know what's to be expected of you. You'll anticipate logistical details and thus be better prepared. Visualize a specific task, or review the entire upcoming day.

See yourself not just doing a task or participating, but doing so with ease, fun, and courage, to get yourself in that mindset.

Get Organized

Gather supplies or ingredients; find files; take preliminary notes—get organized in whatever way makes sense for the task. It doesn't matter how small the task is either (e.g., a call to set up an appointment)—preparing helps.

Create Checklists

Do your best the first few times you do a recurring task—like your taxes or writing up a business newsletter—while creating a step-by-step process list as you go. That way, you never again waste time and generate stress trying to remember how to do it.

Update the list as your process improves, and see how your resistance to starting this task lessens and lessens.

Pause to Refocus

By refocusing, you respond to indecision, stress, doubt, disorganization, or emotional distress in a way that isn't engaging in your BFRB. For example, situations in which to pause and refocus include when you need to:

Prioritize

Maybe having too many possible directions is overwhelming you; get that to-do list or write one now. In what order do these make the most sense? What's the best use of your time in this very moment?

Transition from One Activity to the Next

It can help to pause and refocus between tasks or segments of your day, be it to decompress after the previous activity or to plan for the next.

Brainstorm

Perhaps you're stuck. Pause to brainstorm solutions or ideas.

Vent

Maybe a life problem keeps distracting you. If so, "express your stress" so you can get your head back into whatever you're doing.

◆

It's OK to just stop and contemplate how you're feeling, what you're doing, what you should or could be doing—possibly while playing with a hand-held protector. I can't recommend this enough.

Set Parameters

Start By

When we should be meeting responsibilities and we're not, we can get triggered. We may feel guilt (*I really prefer to do this, but I know I need* to do that . . .) as well as indecision (*When will I start that thing . . . Now? Nah. How about now?*).

Committing to start at a specific time, e.g., 3:15 pm, helps keep triggers at bay. The key is to allow yourself to not worry about that thing, guilt-free, *till* the time you've decided upon.

Finish By

Clear time frames help us focus.

With a vague time frame, i.e., "complete this by the end of the day," you may allow too many distractions and start running out of steam before you broach the finish line, or the task may just feel too daunting.

On the contrary, if you tell yourself you're only working or studying till 6:00 pm, for example, you know you have to finish before then, which will encourage you to focus, while making the task feel more manageable.

The idea is, work only till X time so you don't overwork yourself and so you focus enough to *actually* get it done.

If you disregard the cut-off often, though, it'll mean nothing, so respect it. To the extent possible, re-shuffle the next few days if things do spill over, rather than unfairly dipping into your relaxation time.

◆

While we're on this topic—some of us hyper-focus on activities. If the activity's not productive, we can feel down about ourselves. If it's productive, it might not seem so bad, but we must still take care of ourselves: get some fresh air, get our blood pumping, make time for a healthy meal, and express any stress.

Setting parameters helps with this too.

The Pomodoro Technique

The Pomodoro technique is another way to make tasks feel manageable, approachable, fair—rather than like amorphous blobs that may stretch out forever. The technique goes something like this:

- Set a timer for twenty-five minutes, and **do nothing but focus on your task for that long**.

> *You may want to keep scrap paper nearby for notes, ideas, or to-dos unrelated to what you're doing; jot these down to keep them from distracting you, and return to the task right away; aka, remember to pause to refocus.*

- Once time's up, take a break.

> *Choose limited, predetermined breaks (e.g., "sit outside for ten minutes," "watch one video"), rather than aimless ones (e.g., "just take a break"), as this may derail you and leave you dangerously open to picking.*

- After the break, start the next twenty-five-minute "Pomodoro."

◆

You can also tackle something for the length of just one Pomodoro and call it done, e.g., "I'll tidy up for ten minutes." Suppose your home is a mess, it's stressing you out, but you can't commit to cleaning it all. Make progress by setting a timer.

You can also use this technique to make progress on some looming task that doesn't necessarily have a deadline but that needs to get done, aka, something you can put off but which will cause uncomfortable emotions that you may try to escape, like guilt for not doing it.

Attack it via a few Pomodoros a week or month.

◆

Though you can make the Pomodoro longer or shorter, if too little time is spent on an activity, you never get out of start mode. That is, by the time you're settled into the task, time's up.

By contrast, when you focus on an activity for a while, it's like exercise: it takes time to "warm up," but once you do, you get in the flow and the task becomes easier.

This is also why short, measured breaks are recommended—so you stay focused and in the flow, rather than having to try to get back into it over and over. If you *are* in the flow and don't want to take a break, start the next Pomodoro and keep going.

Do One Thing at a Time

The human brain cannot multitask.[19] What we're actually doing is repeatedly switching our focus, which can wear us out.

The antidote to scattering our energy and becoming stressed is to do *one thing at a time*.

Even while doing the smallest tasks (e.g., pouring a glass of water), I try to be methodical and finish one part of the task smoothly and precisely before moving on to the next (*first this, then that, now this*).

After a while, it starts to feel like dancing, like being in that flow.

◆

A bonus of doing one thing at a time is that we get dopamine hits as we finish something,[20] as opposed to when we take on more and more without giving ourselves the satisfaction of completing anything.

Learn About Troublesome Tasks

Learning about a task (even a little) can relieve stress around it and make it easier, so look up articles, videos, or books about whatever is giving you trouble at work or in your personal projects.

No matter what it is, someone is sharing valuable information on it.

Work in Public

In public, most of us are less likely to pick and more likely to stop once we've started, so as a protector, work in a library, cafe, or some public place. You can do this regularly, as a preventative measure, or on days focusing is extra hard and picking is looming.

If you're a student or freelancer, try it.

Do It the Easy Way

We may do something in a more difficult or complicated way because we don't want to take the time or effort to do it the way we realistically know we should. We do it the lazy way.

You know what I'm talking about: carrying a thousand bags of groceries inside at once, rather than just making two trips; not using the right tool because the right tool is stowed away; standing on tip-toe to water plants and spilling water, or endangering ourselves, to avoid getting the step stool—which by the way is right there.

As these little frustrations meld with others throughout our day, we may end up wanting to escape the tension by picking. So just do it the easy way. Put in the additional bit of effort. It may actually save you time, and it will certainly save you frustration.

Do it for your skin, hair, or nails.

Interpersonal

A way to improve how you work, study, or keep up your home is to talk to the other people in those spaces, with the aim of reducing any undue stress you have.

A few examples:

- Set or trade chores with friends, partners, or kids.
- Tell coworkers how you really feel about projects and workloads, in a direct but friendly way.
- Talk to other parents involved in school or hangouts about more evenly sharing responsibilities like pickups, drop-offs, and group projects, or about whether they can take things off your plate entirely, without it causing undue stress for them, during times where you're booked or could use the extra support.

◆

Sometimes talking to others about these things, or working out the details once you have, is easier said than done, but it's worth it. Envision it, plan it, and then take the leap.

Enjoy What You're Doing

If you're not enjoying it, or aren't looking forward to it, don't do it—get yourself out of it. If you have compelling reasons for doing a task or activity, but you aren't happy about it, try the following.

Commit to What You're Doing

While resistance to a task or obligation makes us want to escape it, committing to it gives us energy. To help you commit, consider:

- Why is it important you do this?
- What are reasons you *want* to do this?
- What can you get out of this that *is* related to something you enjoy or care about?
- How will this help you in the future? Will it give you new skills? A view into how others work? New experiences?
- Can you appreciate this activity because it's a self-care habit—or something you just need to do to protect from your BFRB?
- Can you appreciate this activity because it helps someone else, possibly someone you care about?
- Is the task or activity a big deal? Is it actually so bad, or so hard?

In addition:

- Don't stress about being perfect, or doing it perfectly. Simply agree to do your best.
- Take pride in what you're doing—let it represent you, rather than putting in half your effort. Go all in. No matter how small, or possibly unimportant the task.
- Be present. Being distracted makes tasks harder. Like committing, being present offers us energy. (Remember, tune in to your senses to come into the moment—*what is this task like? how does it sound? feel? smell?*).

The above helps when you're facing resistance, but sometimes it's as easy as a mindset shift—just remembering to enjoy.

Make What You're Doing Pleasant Indirectly

Have pleasant scents, sounds, and sights around on a regular basis—and if not regularly, then call these in when you're trying to make tasks more appealing.

You can also do this when you're feeling down, to uplift yourself.

For example, at my desk, I encourage music (with few lyrics), incense, candles, essential oils, plants, flowers, and little knickknacks. This way, work becomes something I look forward to, or at least have less resistance to.

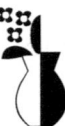

Additional examples of making tasks pleasant indirectly include:

- Watch or listen to YouTube, an audio book, or a podcast while doing chores like washing dishes, folding laundry, or making the bed.
- Listen to audio books or have great music cued up during drives.
- Burn candles and play music while cooking.
- Use soaps, lotions, toothpastes, and more that you actually enjoy, that are a little special, to make these mundane personal hygiene tasks more appealing.
- Make sure you look and smell put together, so you feel better about yourself and in general while doing whatever it is.

•

Making your tasks enjoyable preemptively, as a *foundational habit*, or when you notice resistance, as a *responsive habit*, will help your BFRB immensely.

Your Spaces

Your spaces—your home, dorm, or desk at work—can contribute to how many or how few urges you have. You may have trouble focusing or feel overwhelmed when these are messy and crowded. Conversely, a clean, pleasant space can make you feel bright.

Depending on where you live and work, your space may be harder to manage. Just do your best. Consider these protective tips:

- If an item doesn't have a dedicated place, it'll end up in the way, so create a designated place for *every* item. The keys, the remote, the backpack, the coats, the hats, etc.—*everything in its place*.
- Make your space user-friendly. As best you can, put everything where it'll be most useful and easy to access. Install more hooks, buy space organizers, and move things around till you find the best spots for them.
- Leverage your environment to remind yourself of protectors—e.g., keep hand-held protectors, Band-Aids, head wraps, and other tangible items visible or within reach.
- Choose décor and art that's inspiring to you, reflects who you are at your best, or just makes you happy. You can even create your own.
- Keep your space clean little by little, rather than doing major cleans once everything is out of hand.

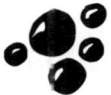

Cleaning, tidying, and organizing help your BFRB in the long-run as *foundational habits*.

They can also be *responsive habits*: Suppose you've forced a break by beginning to scan your scalp or wander toward the mirror—instead choose to tidy up or clean till you re-center and balance out.

> Cleaning and tidying can be soul-cleansing, recalibrating protectors.

Plan Ahead

Yes, iron tonight rather than planning to squeeze it in in the morning; do account for how long it'll take to find parking, and leave a little earlier, rather than winging it; and, of course, fill up the almost-empty water pitcher now, so you have water for later.

In other words, **do things now that'll help you later.**

Applied to any area of your life, this *foundational habit* will help your picking, but it also connects directly to protectors.

Let's say you're going someplace you know you'll be over-stimulated (e.g., a bar, a party, a wedding, a holiday dinner). Before you leave, lay out protective clothing and a journal so they're ready for when you get back. This may be a time to remove mirrors and light bulbs too, to have gloves handy, to make sure you have a healthy meal waiting in the fridge.

Planning ahead can also look like keeping your BFRB in mind when packing for trips—*night-light, fidgets, barriers? Check.*

The message is, anticipate BFRB triggers and set yourself up for success.

Do What You Need to Do for Yourself

Many protectors discussed fall under what I call "doing what you need to do for yourself."

Making the bed so your space feels good, showering because you feel uncomfortable, making food sooner rather than later when hungry, taking the time to re-center when triggered, just getting to bed...

You may not want to, you may not feel like it, you may be *bemoaning* it—but it's what you need to do for yourself, for your BFRB, for your future happiness.

Just do it.

The more you do what you need to do for yourself, the less you'll resist it over time.

More Awareness Tips

Awareness is crucial to healing for many reasons, one of them being that the absolute best time to derail from picking and pulling is *before* getting too caught up in it.

Noticing your hands are searching for targets, retracting them, and then protecting (and celebrating) is part of the rewiring needed to heal. But if you almost never notice when your hands have started roaming, or when you've started pulling, till you, for example, have a pile of hair beside you, additional tools can help deepen your awareness. Below are a few.

Sticky Notes

You might have tried sticky notes in the past, but this isn't like before, where you maybe placed a sticky note somewhere with an encouraging message or warning and expected it to keep you from your skin.

Sticky notes won't get the job done by themselves, but they are great reminders. Put a sticky note, *or some other cue*, in the places you pick so that when your eyes fall on it, you're reminded to check whether you're picking, or angling to.

Use them to remind you to invoke other protectors, like keeping the lights dim or wearing protective clothing or coverings, too.

Alarms

Set alarms for your favorite picking or pulling times, reminding yourself to check whether you're currently engaging in your BFRB, or angling to.

> *Switch up reminders. Once the mind gets used to something, it stops noticing it; it blends into the background. Place reminders in different locations. Vary your wording. Change the time or tone of alerts.*

Bracelets

HabitAware's Keen bracelet buzzes when your hand does whatever action you program the bracelet to notice, such as raise to your scalp or face. This product, combined with other tools, has helped BFRBers.

As a free or cheap alternative, some create their own noisy, heavy bracelet to alert them to potential picking or pulling.

Band-Aids

Rather than covering each individual spot, place a single Band-Aid on a general target area (e.g., a shoulder, your back). When fingertips reach this material, it'll call attention to your behavior, reminding you to pull away and practice a protector.

Hair pullers might place these at the hairline, behind their ears, or at the nape, depending on target areas.

Hair Clips

Place hair clips or bobby pins on your head or hairline. The material will alert you to pull away and check whether you're trying to escape any uncomfortable emotions.

Foundational Blocks

We're nearing the end of More Examples of Protectors, but pay attention, because what's to come is revolutionary for BFRB healing. Remember that the best way to manage urges is to prevent them altogether, as much as possible, and you do that by having a solid foundation. This starts with the basics.

Few of us can withstand a life overhaul; even if we want to, we will not suddenly eat and sleep perfectly or workout like champs.

Only once we stabilize one habit (or a *few*) can we successfully add another.

My intention is to offer ideas for building upon what you already do well, or placing down the first foundational block. We'll be covering:

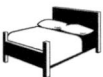

Sleep

While stress, anxiety, depression, and ADHD can negatively affect sleep, the relationship goes both ways—sleep has a *positive* influence on these triggering disorders.[23]

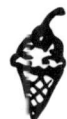

Food

In addition to improving the *look* of skin, hair, and nails (big things for BFRBers), eating right helps skin **heal better and faster**—think scarring and wounds.[24] This is why eating extra healthy after a picking spree is a good idea.

It also encourages hair to **grow faster and stronger**,[25] which is why one hair puller I know of ate healthier at the turning point of her healing, thinking along the same lines.

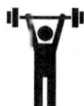

Movement

Increased blood flow is fantastic for the body's biggest organ—the skin (think about when your cheeks thrum as the blood brings nutrients to your face).[26] Movement also de-stresses, relaxes, and helps us sleep/eat better.

◆

Even if you pick up just a few new habits from the following, and I do mean a few, healing will be easier. Let's start with your sleep.

> *If you have preferences or doctor-ordered guidelines that negate any of the below, please disregard it.*

Sleep Better

Get Enough Sleep

You know most adults should be getting seven to nine hours of sleep (teens can get up to ten),[27] but how much sleep do *you* need?

I answered this question for myself by letting my body sleep as much as it wanted to for a few days in a row. The first day, I slept ten hours. The next day, it was eight, and it's been eight on most days since.

Go ahead and let your body sleep for however long it wants to over a long weekend or during a vacation.

> *One or two days of this experiment isn't enough, because the body may sleep longer for a day or more if you've been sleep deprived,[28] which may give you a false idea of how much sleep you need.*

If you can't do this sleep experiment now, safely assume your ideal amount of sleep is at least **seven hours**.[29] Though there are exceptions among us, for most, getting less than seven hours of sleep can seriously affect depression, anxiety, addiction issues, and much more.[30]

One of my many bad sleep habits was that I'd go to bed with no regard for what time I had to be up. Now that I know how much lack of sleep affects me, I have no trouble doing the math to figure out when I must be in bed as it relates to when I must be up, be it for work, school, or some engagement.

I'm a proponent of getting *enough* sleep, even if it means scheduling responsibilities later in the day too, whenever possible.

◆

Planning your life around your sleep may seem like a bit much—until you feel the benefits of it.

Get Consistent Sleep

A key piece to sleep is going to bed and waking up at the same time—even on weekends.[31] (The body doesn't care about the five-day work week that society made up.) This could look like: fall asleep by midnight and wake up at 8:00 am every day.

If you can't realistically do this, even narrowing your sleep window (by keeping your sleep and wake times to within a few hours of each other from day to day) will have you feeling better than a wide, erratic sleep window.

◆

If you're having trouble getting **enough sleep** but can make it so you sleep at **consistent times**—or vice versa—that's a start!

Adjust Your Thoughts

Thoughts, or rather, having too many of them, can keep us awake. If, as the saying goes, *the opposite of sick is healed*, then the opposite of sick here might be:

It's OK to stop directing and forcing my thoughts. I can think about this later. I can just let my thoughts go for right now.

If that's not helping, rather than becoming tangled in a line of thinking, enter a new one: think about whatever book you're reading, whatever show you're watching, or use visualization to enter some made-up, fantastical place in your mind.

If you can't let go, particularly if it's a heavy topic, keep thinking about it, but reframe your thoughts in a more positive or neutral light.

For example, I often stayed up because I was afraid, and I know I'm not alone in this. The opposite of fearful is *safe*. I fostered a feeling of safety by changing my thinking:

I am safe.

I've done the things I need to do, like lock the doors and leave a light on. A loved one, or even a neighbor, is nearby.

I can't control the whole world anyway, so if something bad is going to happen, I'll deal with it then. I'm tough. I'm capable.

◆

Thoughts can also be harnessed to help us wake up.

Often, I'd wake up and immediately feel dread. Or I'd argue with myself: *Why can't you just get up?*

Now I change my thinking, right there in bed, till I feel better:

My tasks will not be that bad. I will enjoy the things I have to do.

I will do one thing, then the next.

All I have to do right now is drink water.

If I get up, I can drink a warm cup of coffee . . .

Or, *I know I didn't sleep enough. Today might be a little hard, but I'm going to try my best and do whatever small things will help me get through it.*

I side with myself and think of whatever I can to (kindly) convince myself to get up. And if I have nothing pressing to do, I give my body the rest it clearly needs.

◆

For those who start picking if they languish in bed, rather than adjusting morning thoughts, even better is to train yourself to jump out of bed *before* thoughts start.

Create Pleasant Mornings

If we have nothing to look forward to, why *would* we want to get up?

My mornings now include lighting a candle for atmosphere while I shower, with music or motivational videos playing through a portable speaker. To make this low-effort, I have my Morning Playlist ready to go.

For you, a morning routine worth looking forward to might start with wearing earbuds in bed, so you don't disturb your partner, and catching up on an audio book; following a guided meditation; or enjoying music you like—for even a few minutes if that's all you can do.

> Build things to look forward to into the future as well: a weeklong vacation somewhere far, or a weekend trip nearby; a concert, play, or show; a movie or game night; a restaurant reservation; or things related to life dreams.

A long, relaxed morning may not be possible on days you work or go to school. However, for the sake of your BFRB, a routine that allows you to get everywhere on time, feeling prepared, needs to be. And even then, small pleasantries can be woven in.

◆

While an *enticing* morning routine may include immediately checking emails or social media, a *pleasant* one probably does not. Personally, I save emails for after breakfast, and I never check social media first thing (or almost at all, honestly—I turn off notifications so I can check it on my time).

If you are a social media person, and you enjoy looking at it in the morning, curate your social media to help you protect. Type in "healthy eating," "relaxation," etc., and follow and subscribe.

Create a BFRB-Friendly Night-Time Routine

A BFRB-friendly night-time routine might include:

Do things like washing your face, brushing teeth, filling the humidifier, and setting alarms long before you reach that uncomfortable space where tiredness has taken over so you want to sleep, but you're not set up for it, so you can't—as this is prime time for picking.

While you still have the energy, make sure you have the right temperature, number of pillows, thickness of blankets, and more. A comfortable bed and room will not only help you fall asleep, but also help keep you asleep. If you do wake up, *adjust* what you need to (e.g., temperature), *do* what you need to (e.g., use the bathroom), and get right back to bed, especially if you pick in the middle of the night.

To make getting to bed more enticing, as part of your routine, make your night-time atmosphere enjoyable. For example, spritz an essential oil over your bed or buy an essential oil diffuser; plug in a Himalayan salt lamp; and play light music or a meditation.

Notice If You Resist Sleep

For most of my life, I pushed sleep off with distractions, including snacking, TV, and not least—skin picking. Eventually, I realized I was resisting sleep.

At some point, I learned that it's OK to be still. To give my body the sleep it's asking for. To leave things for later. It's more than OK. *It's what I need to do for myself.* I learned to discover and address what was keeping me from sleep.

◆

I don't want to minimize potential sleep troubles, but if you can relate, I encourage you to figure out how to help yourself in this area.

There is a way.

And, at times, it may be as simple as noticing whether you're putting off rest for no good reason, and deciding to *just get to sleep.*

While improving your general sleeping pattern is a protective, *foundational habit*, getting to sleep is an in-the-moment, *responsive habit.* If you look at the clock and it's late, getting to bed when you feel like escaping, when you're tired, is just the best thing to do.

Eat Right

Eat More of the Good Stuff

No matter whether you're vegan, vegetarian, pescatarian, or eat whatever, some stuff is not good for us—our looks, mood, health, or **urges**.

Many BFRBers, including me, see a connection between certain foods and increased urges. With exceptions, these include:

- **Processed foods** (much unrefrigerated, pre-packaged, or fast food)
- **Fried foods**
- **Refined grains*** (white pasta, white bread, pizza crust)
- **Refined sugar*** ("added sugars"—pastries, candy, wrapped snacks)

* Aka, simple/refined carbs

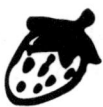

In my experience and in the experience of others, because of the fiber in it, among other reasons,[32] sugar in fruit doesn't have the same effect as processed, added sugar, on BFRBs.

Eating less of the above will very likely mean fewer sessions.

That's incredible. That said, trying to *not* eat these can be hard, so eat more of the good stuff instead. The idea is to focus on healthfulness (*eat this*), rather than on deprivation (*don't eat that*).

Depending on your diet or needs, the good stuff might mean:

- **Fruits & vegetables** (e.g., spinach, broccoli, plantains, berries)
- **Whole grains** (e.g., oats, quinoa, bulgur, brown rice)
- **Nuts & seeds** (e.g., pumpkin seeds, sunflower seeds, cashews)
- **Probiotic-rich foods** (e.g., kimchi, miso)

- **Well-sourced fish or meat** (e.g., grass-fed, wild-caught)
- **Legumes** (e.g., beans, lentils)

Here are small but tangible ways to reduce urges via a better diet if you have trouble in this area:

- **Eat one naturally green thing a day.** When I learned that leafy vegetables are the most nutrient-rich things we can eat (i.e., disease-protecting and life-extending),[33] I committed to doing this. I counted anything from a side of broccoli to a few lettuce leaves in a sandwich. (I'd write "Eat 1 green thing" in my to-do list to remind myself.)

    I now easily eat and enjoy large lunch salads. When you eat more of the good stuff, something you can look forward to is that you crave the junk less.[34]

- **Eat a healthy breakfast no matter what.** For me this means the first thing I eat in the day cannot be junk, though I can eat the junk after. Sometimes, I do; other times, I don't crave it anymore.

    Perhaps for you keeping dinner healthy is easier.

- **Don't compromise taste for health** often, or you won't keep up with your healthy eating habits for long. Find a way to season or prepare the food in a way you actually like.

Drink More of the Good Stuff

It's not just about what you eat. Drinks to avoid or minimize include:

- **Soda**
- **Fruit juice** with added sugar

Again, trying to *not* drink these will be hard, so replace unhealthy drinks with healthier ones like:

- **Green or white tea** (these help build collagen, something many pickers want!)
- **Herbal tea** (chamomile, hibiscus, lavender, or any of the endless, gorgeous, aromatic options)
- **Seltzer** (so many flavors out there—watermelon, cherry, peach, blueberry, coffee)
- **Water**

Mind Your Booze Intake

Another drink to look out for if you're a BFRBer: alcohol.

Many see a correlation between excess alcohol and not only pimples but also sessions.

When you're drunk, not giving in to picking or pulling can be even harder. When you're hungover, you may be low, and physically stressed, and have fresh new pimples on top of that. And these are just a few reasons alcohol may affect BFRBers.

If alcohol is affecting your BFRB, is it worth it to cut back?

If nothing else, *note* whether it makes a difference in your picking. The more information we have, the more empowered we are to make changes, even if it's not right away.

Don't Get Too Hungry

Am I hungry? It's not always easy to tell, but it becomes easier once you start paying attention. If you're craving a snack or junk in the middle of the day, even if you don't *feel* hungry, that's one sign.

Getting a little hungry is nothing to be scared of, and fasting has tons of benefits.³⁵ But it's one thing to do this intentionally and in an informed way, and another to have an erratic eating schedule that leaves you feeling out of sorts.

To avoid getting too hungry, think about **what** you'll eat, and **when**, ahead of time.

Don't Eat Too Much or Too Little

If you eat too little in one sitting, you'll be hungry before long, and possibly triggered.

If you eat too much, you'll be lethargic, and possibly triggered.

Finding out your ideal portions takes practice. Till then, here's a protector I use that you may like: Save food when you're full—yes, even if it's a few bites (that's why tiny Tupperware exists).

Balance Your Meals

A balanced meal includes the three macro-nutrients: healthy fats, protein, and complex carbs.

If thinking in terms of balanced meals makes sense to you, do so. It's a great idea for your health and urges. However, if it stresses you out or doesn't make sense yet, just eat a large variety of the good stuff.

Keep Blood Sugar Stable

When blood sugars rocket or dip drastically—**urges increase**. Earlier I mentioned eating poorly can result in sluggishness and thus the desire to escape. This is one effect of blood sugars being out of whack. Much of what I've discussed above is aimed at keeping your blood sugars stable, but I wanted to say it outright in case you understand blood sugar and find it useful to see it this way.

Try an Elimination Diet for Blemishes and More

Dairy, sugar, gluten, and alcohol (which tends to have gluten) cause breakouts and physical discomfort for some. During an elimination diet, you cut out a suspect food, or type of food, for **two weeks to a month** and note the results. Because of what I've witnessed with my own skin and heard from others, I recommend starting with dairy if you're curious to see whether what you're eating is behind your blemishes.

Some dairy, such as well-sourced goat cheese, may be an exception,[36] so there's hope for cheese lovers.

But at first, fully eliminate dairy. That means cutting out *all* dairy, including less obvious ingredients like casein and whey, so get to know your labels. The "all" is important: if you're not consistent, you may get confusing results, which won't be helpful.

As mentioned, if you primarily pick at blemishes, having *few to no blemishes* will help you manage your excoriation immensely.

Treat Right

Treats are a simple pleasure of life. To enjoy this simple pleasure while being mindful of your BFRB, try the following:

- *Make* your own desserts or pastries, to make sure they're healthi*er*, e.g., replace certain ingredients with healthier, more BFRB-friendly alternatives.
- Snack on fruit. Yes, fruit you truly enjoy—for me, mangos make the world go round—can become a replacement for junk food, especially if you're committed to healing your BFRB.

The idea is, if you're going to snack anyway, possibly at a crazy hour, it might as well be something healthy, whether or not it's fruit specifically.

- Pair refined carbs (e.g., a white bagel, pancakes, or cookies) with whole fruit to blunt the blood sugar spike.[37]
- Pair refined carbs (e.g., white rice, pasta, or bread) with plant-based fats or proteins (e.g., nuts, avocado, almond butter) to blunt the blood sugar spike.[38]

To make this simple, ignore the above and just eat less-than-ideal items alongside a balanced meal. (They were on to something with dessert.)

- Opt for the lesser evil (e.g., choose non-dairy ice cream if dairy causes breakouts, aka, pick the snack that triggers you or your acne *less*).
- If you *are* going to eat the worst of the junk, keep it to small doses, whether it be buying, making, or serving yourself smaller portions.

◆

Okay, let's say you over-did it.

Your thoughts won't replace minding the basics, but they can support you. For example, rather than bemoaning, *I ate a lot of sugar, which means I'm going to pick!* You can think, *I ate a lot of sugar, but thankfully I'm aware this is a trigger. I'm going to be extra diligent with protectors.*

Thoughts can also help you beforehand. For example, play out the scenario. Imagine yourself eating the junk, all the way through, past the good part. Do you still want it as much?

Eating cookies till I have a stomach ache seems to be the kind of person I am. No matter how much I tell myself that I'll eat a few now and save some for later. Now that I've acknowledged it and stopped scolding myself for it, I see the humor in it, and I just do what I need to do to for myself: buy them only rarely and make them myself only here and there, in small batches.

Trust me, I love junk food—but I love feeling and looking great, having energy, and reduced urges more.

Recognize What You're Actually Eating

As with skin picking itself, awareness is a step to eating right. Track what you eat for *even a week* to help you be objective. It's as easy as jotting it in a journal, a note app, or an app like MyFitnessPal.

If this seems like too much, do just this one thing: see how you feel **after you eat**. This is a great way to judge whether certain foods ramp up urges.

Move Some

Don't Exercise

"Exercise" has the connotation of going somewhere special (e.g., the gym) and carving out dedicated time for an isolated activity. But especially if you aren't aiming for a bigger this or smaller that and only want to be healthier and ease BFRB urges, simply incorporate more movement into your life.

Try the following:

Hiking and gardening do double-duty. They not only offer movement, but by connecting us with nature, they can alleviate depression[39] and feelings that lead to picking.

If you don't have a garden, or a patch you can turn into one, taking care of potted plants can be your form of gardening.

To find trails for hiking, type your city into the AllTrails app (download it now if this interests you).

> *Remember to wear sunscreen, proper clothing/shoes, and bug spray (bonus, the fewer bug bites, the fewer reasons to touch your skin).*

Yoga combines movement and attention given to the self to become an overall feel-good, stress-relieving experience that goes beyond exercise. It can be modified for all levels (chair yoga is a thing).

I like to grab a mat, set up YouTube on my TV or laptop, and follow along to a video that's anywhere from five to twenty-five minutes long.

> *Yoga is wonderful for those times when nothing you try is bringing relief or peace emotionally.*

If you don't like yoga, or want variety, look into the "moving meditation" **qigong**.

Dancing is one of my favorite ways to move more. It's ancient. It's human. It raises endorphins and reduces the stress hormone cortisol.[40]

Dance for the length of one song or longer: get silly, without judgment of yourself, or get good at it, if you want.

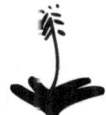

Cleaning or tidying up is movement in its own right. Enjoy and appreciate every step and bend, and the accompanying sweat and heavy breathing. It's good for you and, thus, for your BFRB.

◆

As a *foundational habit*, practice one or more of the above routinely. As a *responsive habit*, pick one to do when you feel like escaping.

> *While these get you moving, they're also absolutely ways to relax, rejuvenate, or balance out.*

◆

Lastly, you can also sneak movement into the mundane. For example, don't drive around looking for the closest parking spot; in fact, park far.

Rather than take the elevator, choose the stairs every time they're an option.

Going for a coffee? Walk there.

How can you work more movement into your life?

Notice How Your Muscles Feel

Muscles can feel loose, tight/tense, or fine. Move some to reduce the chances of BFRB sessions that may be around the corner.

Does any part of your body feel tight or tense? If yes, relax via:

- Stretching (don't force it; savor it)
- Massage (from yourself or a loved one)

> Even little massages and squeezes add up. This is a great protector! If you're going to massage yourself, though, avoid fingertips on target areas. Use your knuckles or massage tools, or do it over clothes.

- Conscious relaxation of the tense areas (we can habitually hold tension in our shoulders, neck, brow, and chin—consciously relaxing takes practice, and at times, it can be difficult; if you find you chronically *can't* relax tense muscles, look into progressive muscle relaxation)

Do your muscles feel weak or uncomfortable (kind of . . . loose)? If the answer is yes, "tighten" muscles by:

- Doing a few push-ups
- Squeezing the "loose" areas
- Doing yoga

◆

Barring serious physical ailments, if something specific is bothering you, look up exercises online. For example, many of us have back or neck pain that isn't related to some underlying medical problem, and which can be ameliorated with just a little effort.

And if physical conditions do keep you from certain movements, do what you can, and again, be shamelessly proud.

Small Actions

Little efforts may not seem worth it. It may feel like you might as well do nothing. But *doing something*, consistently, is how we grow.

Doing, say, five squats or push-ups every other day won't get you to your body goals, and it may not significantly reduce urges.

But do those five squats.

And if light stretching in the morning, in bed or right next to your bed, is all you can manage, that's great.

In fact, be shamelessly proud of these small efforts, *especially* if you do them consistently, because only once these are established will you have a foundation to build upon.

◆

Once you have a small action down, you may feel so good you'll want to take on the world. And you may be able to. But if committing to too much has now made you want to do nothing, it means your foundation wasn't solid enough yet.

Backtrack, make the action small again, and build little by little.

Move Every Twenty Minutes

Our bodies want to *move,* so if you find it's been twenty minutes or more since you last moved, walk the perimeter of your office or home; do a few squats in the bathroom at work. If you can't or don't want to stand, at least twist your spine (gently); rotate your ankles; look over each shoulder for a few; or activate certain muscles (e.g., squeeze your glutes or do a Kegel).

Twenty minutes is a rule of thumb. It doesn't have to be exact.

Remove Obstacles

Obstacles get in the way of protective habits.

To remove resistance, remove obstacles. When it comes to more movement, this can look like:

🚧 OBSTACLE

Unsure what to do—no plan or don't know much about fitness

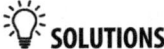 **SOLUTIONS**

Identify your goals to help guide you.

Learn exercises and routines by following videos.

Write your routines out (on paper or in your note app).

Work with a trainer.

🚧 **OBSTACLE**
Not enough space to work out at home

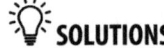 **SOLUTIONS**

Move stuff so you have more room.

Go outside or go to a gym.

Modify your moves so you can do them in the space you have.

🚧 **OBSTACLE**
Not fun

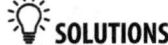 **SOLUTIONS**

Don't "exercise" (see earlier section).

Remind yourself *why* you're doing it, to keep you going even when it's not fun.

Attach a cellphone mount near exercise equipment so you can watch a show while working out.

🚧 **OBSTACLE**
Too much setup

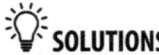 **SOLUTIONS**

Prioritize movement by keeping workout equipment out/setup/open and making sure nothing is put on top of it; this way, you can do a few reps whenever you feel inspired, rather than letting the inspiration be sapped by all the setup.

Sleep with workout clothes on, or with them right next to your bed, to make working out in the morning easier.

Challenge Yourself

Some of us crave a challenge more than we know. Be careful with your body, but also realize how capable it is. Our bodies can do incredible things and achieve feats: marathons, free climbing, tight-rope walking, gymnastics, Strongman competitions.

Some challenge, like the Hundred Pushups Challenge, where you train yourself to be able to do one hundred consecutive push-ups in less than two months, might be the incentive you need to move more.

Another idea—make it your goal to be able to do a split if you can't already. The Splits Training app offers a stretching program to get you there.

Or, finally get into that sport or dance that's been in the back of your mind, or try one, like boxing or ballet, that you haven't considered, but that you may enjoy.

Even researching costs and locations is a step.

Bring It All Together with Routines

We all have routines: what we usually do at a certain time. That's what a routine is. But these routines aren't always intentional; they don't always help us.

Intentional routines are beneficial for BFRBers for two main reasons:

1

They create space for the habits that help us manage urges. Just a few examples from above are:

- Relaxation

- Setting parameters (e.g., so you don't study or work too little or too much)
- Things related to the basics (aka, how and when you sleep, eat, and move)
- Beauty and personal care

2

They cut down on aimlessness and indecision. When aimless or indecisive, we're more likely to wander into a session.

When you're unsure what to do next, consider what's next in your intentional routine—it certainly isn't picking or pulling.

◆

Routines can have the connotation of being boring, but:

- You can build **options** into your routine.

Novelty produces dopamine,[41] so switching it up keeps routines from getting stale too.

- You can weave **pleasantness** into your routine.

The things you do on the average day make up your life so make the mundane things pleasant.

- A routine doesn't take away the potential for **spontaneity**; just adjust it as the day calls for it.

Being aimless and scattered or rushing at certain points of the day isn't spontaneous anyway.

◆

Structure is protective for BFRBers, so create or enhance existing routines. To help you, I recommend the following.

Be Realistic

To increase your chances of actually sticking to a routine, it must be plausible given *who you are right now*. Though big, sudden changes like going cold turkey or going all in can stick when we're desperate for, or inspired toward, change, easing in is often more realistic.

For example, if you want to watch less TV, limit yourself to, say, two episodes. Write this in your routine. Yes, write in some TV (or gaming—two matches; or social media—ten minutes of scrolling).

This is more realistic than attempting to watch no TV after doing it every night for years.

> Again, in moderation, TV, gaming, social media, and the like can be de-stressing anyway.

From there, include just a little bit of reading, fitness, meditation, time spent on passion projects, or whatever pertains to *who you'd like to be*.

♦

Choosing a time of day and location is key to getting yourself to do something consistently, as is deciding what you're actually going to do.

Let's take the earlier example of novel-writing. No one just *writes a novel*. Making time to sit at a desk around 8:00 pm to write, say, 300 to 1,000 words, five days a week, is how a 60,000-plus-word novel actually gets written.

Another example is choosing a specific exercise or yoga routine (maybe from YouTube) that you'd like to try, as well as a time and day of the week it might be feasible to do it.

In Foundational Blocks, I recommended doing just a few push-ups every other day to offer you something to build on. This could be included in a routine too.

♦

Now that you've set some realistic goals, implement one or two of them and keep up with just those changes for a few weeks.

As you get more and more comfortable with your routine, add more items, or slowly increase the amount of time you offer to certain items.

Before you know it, you'll have a novel, or an exercise routine you actually do.

Make Time for Yourself

Don't make it so you have to finish all your tasks before you get to do what you'd *like* to, or what you *need* to do for yourself to be BFRB-free.

Because you'll never finish.

Something will *always* come up. Another project. Another to-do.

You'll have to actively make time for joy, decompression, movement, trips to nature, visiting friends, and passion projects. And we are more likely to do these things when we make time for them in our routines.

I learned that to be more productive (and keep BFRB urges low) I can't afford *not* to take time for myself. In other words, allowing relaxation and fun makes us *more productive*, with work, school, and other responsibilities . . . It allows us to work better and faster and want to escape less, so making time for ourselves is far from frivolous, no matter how many items are on our to-do list.

Know That Your Routine Can Change

Your routine may shift throughout the year, or the week, depending on responsibilities. Also, your routine for work days may look different than for days off. That's OK.

Be flexible in the face of whatever's going on at different points in your life (going to school, taking care of a baby, competing). Go with the seasons as well as your own cycles, your highs and lows.

Hit the Touchstones

Often, when we're most tempted to throw out routines and other things that keep us grounded is when we most need them.

I'd chuck my entire routine when I felt I didn't have enough time, but I learned that touching upon my routine's most important points—even if they're *condensed*—is essential. After all, these points involve protective habits.

So, for example, if you can't have the long, luxurious morning you like to, at least hit the most important items. If some things do need to be cut altogether on some days, try not to let it be those protective touchstones that keep you grounded and sane.

Not to mention, hitting the touchstones allows you to keep the intentional routine you worked so hard for in place, rather than letting it devolve back into your possibly not-so-helpful, default routine.

Adjust Your Routine so It Works Better

You may notice some parts of your routine never get done or that they start to fall by the wayside. That means it's time to modify.

Some ideas:

- **Shift the time you do something** to a little earlier or a little later. Or move things from your night routine to your morning routine and vice versa.

- **Switch it up.** Change something about this part of your routine. Try new exercises, ingredients, hobbies, locations, products, etc., to keep it novel.

- **Analyze and remove obstacles.** What's making this annoying to do? What's causing resistance?

- **Make it smaller.** Have resistance to meditating for five minutes? Try three minutes.

If you create some small bite and still have resistance to it, make it even smaller. But you must then **commit** *to that small bite. At a certain point, you just have to do it.*

- **Refocus and recommit.** Maybe you lost the thread. Why did you want this in your routine again? What's your goal? What are you trying to accomplish? Remind yourself.

Routines may not be achieved perfectly every day or week, but if we do most things most of the time, we're that much happier and **less likely to crave to escape.**

I highly recommend bringing together all that we've discussed with intentional routines.

A Final Word on Step 3

With your increased awareness of what causes you to pick, you have the power to protect from *each and every* one of those triggers.

Because they are as varied as the triggers they correspond with, protectors come in many forms. If it protects you from picking (in a healthy or benign way)—it's a protector.

I cannot give the answer to how to protect in every situation. But the above has helped me and innumerable others. BFRBers with your specific body-focused repetitive behavior are a fountain of ideas for protectors (though they likely won't call them "protectors"). Search places like YouTube, Reddit, and online forums for more ideas.

♦

With what you've just learned, you can go far, but to save you from unneeded frustration, Step 4 has the finer points on how to use protectors to guard against your BFRB.

You're almost there.

Congratulations on any and all progress you've made with your BFRB up to this point!

Step 4

Practice Protectors

Why Practice Matters

While in the last step you got to know protectors and were encouraged to brainstorm and list yours, this step is about applying them.

You will not be excellent with protectors all the time. You will forget or outright *defy* them. Protectors are new to you, while your BFRB has compelled you for a long time. However, over time, you can master your protectors.

And mastering protectors means healing.

The following concepts take the basic message (*trigger meet protector*) to the next level.

How to Practice Protectors

Some of these concepts have been introduced but are worth repeating. Others are completely new.

> As you read on, please keep logging, identifying triggers, and brainstorming your own protectors.

Work with What You've Got

Because there are so many options, to heal you don't *need* any one thing, e.g., a night-light, a worry stone, a new journal, a fidget or sensory toy—certainly not programmable lights. It may help, but it's far from make or break.

Get creative to start healing right away.

For example, go outside to find a smooth rock, repurpose an already-half-filled journal, or make your own protectors with household items.

This doesn't mean don't protect from *every* trigger; just that you can be flexible in how you do it.

Congratulate Yourself

When you protect in any way, congratulate yourself.

Ideally, you'll do this every time.

As I said, celebrating isn't just a nice thing to do. It rewires you.

Celebrating or congratulating yourself tells your brain **to do what it just did again**, in this case, to protect, because doing so felt good!

This might be one of the most important points in this guide, because without it, protectors may not stick.

A BFRB becomes part of one's life due to the simple habit loop which all humans are susceptible to:

$$\text{Cue} \rightarrow \text{Behavior} \rightarrow \text{Reward}$$

To make protectors stick, we must use the same habit loop. (This loop is how *all* habits are made and broken.)

While the cue, aka whatever is triggering us, will often stay the same, our **new behavior** is protecting (rather than picking), and our **new reward** is celebrating (rather than that release, satisfaction, stimulation, etc., from picking).

Leveraging this habit loop by intentionally celebrating, rather than leaving it to chance whether we feel good after protecting, is how we wire in these new, better behaviors—aka protectors—solidly and more quickly.

So, to celebrate, smile; dance a little; dust your shoulders off; take a peaceful breath; offer yourself some treat or reward; verbally or mentally congratulate yourself ("Go me!")—do whatever you feel like doing in the moment as you savor your success.

In practice, this might look like retracting your hand from a target, taking a deep breath as you hold adhi mudra, while smiling at yourself because you've protected.

◆

Anytime you keep from picking or pulling, that's one session avoided. Clearer skin and fuller hair ahead! Plenty of reason to be happy and satisfied with yourself. It's time to focus on your successes just as much as—if not much more—than you ever have your failures. For many reasons, not least because it's part of healing.

As a shortcut, just remember to **act**:

Acknowledge the urge or trigger, **C**ounter it, and then be **T**hankful you did.

Harness Go-To Actions

Protectors come in many forms, and go-to actions are an important one. Remember, a **go-to action** is something you do immediately after derailing a precursor or stopping yourself from picking or pulling.

It's like a parachute you activate as you see the cliffside and know you're about to go over. It carries you safely to the ground.

In this section we'll cover a few ways to harness go-to actions. First, here are some of the go-tos we discussed. When you notice you've been picking, or when you realize you're about to, **immediately**:

- Snap or clap.
- Cradle your thumb(s) in adhi mudra.
- Fold your hands.
- Take a deep breath.
- Grab a hand-held protector or fidget.
- Stimulate one of your senses (for ideas, see earlier section).
- Tune in to your senses (i.e., ground yourself).
- Press your lips together (instead of chewing your cheeks).

Go-tos can be combined. For example, practice adhi mudra while taking a deep breath.

◆

To take this further, focus on the go-to action, if possible (with some, this might not make sense). For example, if you chose a hand-held protector, *what does the object look or feel like?* If you chose to stimulate your senses, *what does this thing look, feel, smell, sound, or taste like?*

Ideally, you'll focus on the go-to for a minute plus. If you can't commit to a minute, focus on it at least **till the immediate urge has passed.** And, of course, congratulate yourself during, or after.

◆

Your go-to may depend on the current situation and location, so brainstorm a few go-tos you can practice in each of the main picking locations you've identified, e.g., toilet, desk, car, in bed, in front of the TV.

I recommend listing potential go-tos in your Protectors List now. Adapt them to better suit you as you practice.

In these favorite BFRB locations, **being proactive is still best**, especially if you're someone who rarely notices your behavior till way after it's started. For example, if you've realized you pull while watching movies, adjust your position on the couch and have protectors in hand (e.g., a fidget) before the movie even starts. If you pick on the toilet, hold adhi mudra as you sit.

By doing this, go-tos will come automatically when you *do* need them to derail a precursor to your picking, pulling, or biting.

◆

Choose at least *one* go-to action to try if you haven't already. If you use your hands for your behavior, I highly recommend adhi mudra or snapping, though, truthfully, a go-to action can be *anything* you do to zap the forward momentum toward picking, pulling, or biting. You can even make something up on the spot.

Rather than do any of the go-tos above, I'll sometimes do whatever wacky or funny thing occurs to me to help break the spell and back away in that moment.

As I've said, the longer we engage in precursors, the more the compulsion to pick or pull ramps up. Put differently, the more momentum we have, the harder it is to turn back. So, at the edge, the most important thing is to **just respond.** Aka, practice the first go-to action that comes to mind, right away.

You may not have the capacity to enact a go-to, if you're too consumed by an urge. This is normal. But keep trying. You'll be glad when you do prevent sessions in this way.

◆

This may not make perfect sense till you try it. But before long, you'll be averting your eyes and retracting your hands as unconsciously as you used to give in to picking, applying a go-to at just the *thought* of touching or looking.

Protect Big, Small, and In Between

I singled out go-to actions because they apply in those crucial moments *right* before a session, but a go-to action won't always be enough to keep you from picking or pulling.

It's not that go-tos aren't excellent; it's just that all protectors have their time and place.

For example, you realize you're lightly engaging in precursors, but you don't feel particularly triggered. You're feeling fine.

Or, yes, you're *mildly triggered*, but you want or need to push yourself a bit in your current task.

In this case, practice some small protector, such as repeating a mantra, discharging the discomfort with a breath, grabbing a worry stone, changing into a more protective shirt, covering a blemish with a bandage, or tying your hair so it stops tickling your face and making you scratch and search for bumps.

Congratulate yourself.

Then return to whatever you were doing.

This is just a bit of steady rewiring. No harm done. Sometimes, a small protector is all it takes.

◆

But don't ignore a growing desire to escape.

Repeatedly trying to pick, pull, or bite, even once you've enacted a go-to or applied some other small protector, is a signal that it's time to protect in a bigger way.

Maybe that means stopping what you're doing to eat, taking a break to regroup, journaling to change your mindset, doing a breathing exercise right where you are, or just getting to sleep. It depends on what you're trying to escape from—on what you need—but the point is, if you're decently triggered and the feeling is only mounting, a go-to, a barrier, or some small responsive habit **will not be enough**, and you'll likely pick, pull, or bite.

Yes, stopping everything to journal or make a meal does take more effort, but effort and self-care is what healing body-focused repetitive behaviors often calls for.

◆

There's no hard or fast rule. But if I find myself with roaming hands that I have to pull away *three* times within a short span (or I'm engaging in precursors repeatedly throughout the day, e.g., continuing to flick on the bathroom light to randomly groom or "just look" at myself), I recognize I'm on the brink of picking, and I protect in some larger way as soon as possible.

Check In Often

By checking in with yourself frequently, you'll learn to recognize when you're being triggered in the first place.

You'll also catch triggers and urges when they're small. The smaller they are, the more manageable, which means you have a greater chance of successfully protecting.

Try checking in now. Many "windows" can indicate how you're doing, such as:

- Your breathing (is it shallow, deep, or normal—are you holding your breath?)
- Your heart rate (is it fast, slow, or normal?)
- Your muscles (are they tight, loose, or normal?)
- Your stomach (is it tight, hungry, overly stuffed, knotted from stress, or neutral?)
- Your thoughts (are they clustered and negative, or are you clear-headed, positive, fine?)
- Do you have any pain?

- Your posture (are you slouched or straight?)
- Your speed (are you anxiously rushing, lethargic and slow, or neutral?)
- Steadiness (are you steady or shaky?—shakiness might indicate nervousness, being overly caffeinated, or hunger)

After some practice, you'll learn which windows give you the best indication of how you're doing.

At this point, I don't consciously check these windows. I'm attuned to myself and can just tell how I'm doing. If signals are coming up that I'm unbalanced, I may ask myself:

How am I doing?
Do I need anything?

♦

Being someone who needs a lot of balancing out doesn't make you incapable or weak, though it can feel like that sometimes, especially in the beginning. It can be frustrating. By taking control of your wellbeing and checking in, though, you're showing just how capable you are.

Especially if you're used to bypassing your needs and emotions with your BFRB, it can take practice to recognize and acknowledge these needs and emotions. By continuing to pay attention, though, you'll notice the shifting winds early and let that determine what you do next, how you can protect.

♦

Once you have protected, see how you feel. Do you need to do more, or was what you did enough to erase the trigger or bring the urge down?

In other words, check in again.

Be Responsive

Several triggers can be present at once, so protecting might often look like this:

Find a worry stone (*because hands have started roaming*) and carry it around as you set up a fan (*because you're hot, which is distracting you*). After that, eat (*because you missed lunch and can't focus*) and then recite some mantras (*because you feel pressured by everything you have to get done today*).

Finally, make green tea (*because you ate as a protector, but you accidentally ate too much, and now you're sleepy*), etc.

With practice, addressing triggers will be like a dance. You'll remain positive and in the flow as you do what you need to do for yourself, easily figuring out what that is, or approaching it like a welcome puzzle—*with curiosity*—trying one thing then the next till you get it right. You'll respond fluidly and proactively, moment by moment, bringing yourself back to balance as many times as it takes. Sometimes, it'll be this easy.

Some days, it'll be hard.

Suppose you have several triggers, and they're growing. You feel overwhelmed. You want to protect, but you're not sure what to do.

This is a good time to "pause to refocus." You can do this in several ways. One is to grab scrap paper and write down whatever current triggers come to mind, plus what you can do about them.

For example:

Hungry?	Snack on nuts while making lunch
Hot!	Put the fan closer; move into a cooler room?
Tired	Drink green tea
I have a project due today!	You have time. It's early in the day. Just do your best.

◆

When you're triggered but aren't sure how or what to do about it, you can also pause and log. You don't have to wait to have an outright **urge** to log. After all, triggers lead to urges.

Even if you know how to protect, consider logging *anyway*. You may discover a better or additional protector.

Look Beyond the Target

Sure, you're no longer going out of your way just to scrutinize, but if you happen to notice something tempting, you feel you have to get it, if eventually. So, are you really healing?

This was my doubt at the start of healing, and it may be yours too. But remember what I said earlier:

The desire to escape is the bigger force.

Ever notice you *can* sometimes keep a session from going too far? You pick or pull just a few things, and then you stop.

Compare this to when you pick anything accessible, leaving untouched only tiny, difficult spots, and/or targets on "forbidden" areas you *really* want to leave alone.

Compare *that* to when you go for anything you can possibly reach, scouring your body, no matter how tiny, difficult to get, or forbidden.

If it were simply about the target, you'd go for each target no questions asked. But as you can see, it's variable.

You'll still prefer something pickable or pullable *not* be there, but if you're centered, any desire/urge will be much easier to handle. This craving only grows, or becomes unmanageable, **as what we crave to escape grows.**

◆

For me, when the desire to *get it out* or have it *gone* becomes overwhelming, it's a signal that I've been ignoring triggers, bulldozing them.

I have not been checking in.

I'm not caring about what I eat, my sleep, or whether I get my blood pumping; I'm not taking breaks and relaxing via meditation, yoga, or journaling.

Or if I am, I'm not doing enough; I need to do more, because maybe something big is going on in my life at that time.

> The intensity with which you want to pick or
> pull has to do with your current emotions
> or state, *not* with any BFRB target.

Your BFRB isn't a separate, unfortunate thing happening within your life; it's connected to everything else in your life.

As you stare down a target, if you remember that it's not about that hair or pimple, you might not be as compelled as you were before. Remind yourself that you're better off figuring out or acknowledging what you're trying to escape, *what you need to do for yourself*, instead.

> *Ideally, by keeping barriers and other protectors in place, you won't get close enough to targets to be tempted, not as much as before anyway, but as you practice, you may.*

Despite me saying this, you may feel like it really is about the blemish or hair or skin, like you can't keep your hands off long enough to let anything heal and go away on its own, like you eventually have to pull that hair or scab. But as you practice healthier, more rewarding ways to deal (such as those described under More Examples of Protectors), you'll see you can let blemishes dry up or let that hair or scab or piece of skin be.

You really can.

And when triggers are low, you'll be able to do so *easily*, because, again, it's not really about the target at all.

(You could say it's about triggers. And how do we handle those? We protect. Go back to More Examples of Protectors and your own Protectors List for ways to do this.)

◆

The fact that it's *not* about the target is good news. It means once you get past whatever you want to escape, or meaningfully protect, the urge will drop.

And you won't need to pick or pull for that to happen.

When you do have a tempting target, though, especially when you're new at this and aren't sure how to protect, *take it a day at a time*.

It's a cliché, but it's also great advice for anyone recovering from anything. Even if never picking again for the rest of your life is the goal, it starts with making it to the end of today.

Learn from the Failures

During this process you may feel like you always "forget" to protect, or like you just can't get yourself to.

The thing to do may be to remind yourself to protect next time. Since this is all so new, this is part of practicing.

However, if you *keep* picking in the face of some trigger and *keep* defying or ignoring the corresponding protectors, don't get stuck.

It's time to reassess.

The first few protectors you try may simply not be the best ones. For example, to keep from picking in the middle of the night when I got up to pee, I brainstormed these protectors:

- Place a T-shirt near the bed to wear into the bathroom, or grab my partner's robe.
- Remind myself to not look or touch.
- Keep the lights dim.

But over and over, I didn't *want* to put on the rough T-shirt. I figured a robe, even if it was my partner's, was as good as it got, but it was never in the same spot, so I'd forget to grab it. Despite reminding myself to not look or touch, I'd ruminate over a spot till I became compelled enough to flick the light on so I could get a closer look.

After picking one night too many, I knew I had to try something else. So I bought a robe of my own. It's soft, making it a pleasant protector, and I keep it in the same spot, so it's reasonable to commit to wearing it *every time* I wake up in the middle of the night.

The robe, along with the dim lighting, makes not looking or touching easier. If I had remained stuck, and not adjusted or tweaked, I would've missed out on this effective protector but not on the many night-time sessions I've since avoided.

♦

When I kept finding myself in front of the mirror, I worried the mirror was a trigger I'd never be able to overcome, despite the success I was having protecting from *other* triggers.

Only once I broke it down (rather than staying stuck) could I really protect. What I realized is that I was looking in the mirror even more than usual because I was exploring face yoga, facial massage, correct body and tongue posture, different skin products, and different curly-hair-care methods.

I burrowed down into the chain of events and found the issue wasn't just the mirror but the thoughts that led me to it: *Are these new products working? Is the face yoga working? Let me go look in the mirror . . .*

Not only that, but I'd start wondering about my hair, or skin, or face, as a way to escape, suddenly wanting to check or look because I, unknowingly, craved a distraction.

Now I protect by reminding myself that, *Changes aren't going to happen right away, so checking every few minutes is pointless*—a counter thought.

Also, like anything else, I do the mirror activities listed above in dim lighting—a barrier—rather than letting them become exceptions. I also consciously avoid these mirror activities altogether on days I'm stressed.

> *Stressful days may include when you have "one of those days," when you have an argument, when you're out and about all day, when a project is due, when work or school drained you.*

◆

To offer a final example, here's what I tried in order to be able to pluck my eyebrows in a protected way:

- Switch to brow razors (rather than using one of my favorite picking tools, tweezers).
- Cover blemishes with hydrocolloid bandages in dim lighting, and *only* then, turn on the light to groom brows.
- Groom earlier in the day (because the majority of my picking happened at night, it was worth a shot).
- Groom only before going out (since I wouldn't want to be raw and red for whatever the engagement was).
- Groom only with someone else nearby.
- Groom only on low-stress days.

Some of these worked for a bit on their own, but now I *layer* the best ones: I use an eyebrow razor, and I *may* groom when I'm alone, but mostly only before some event or outing. Overall, I do my eyebrows much less too—only when I need to, not at whim several evenings a week like I used to (which often led to picking . . .).

If I'm thinking about doing my brows at night, particularly when I should be in bed, I remind myself it may be my way of seeking an escape; I may be stressed and not perceiving it, so I'm better off getting to bed or doing something relaxing instead.

◆

If you keep picking, keep **tweaking protectors and dissecting triggers**. Your log and lists are made for this.

This also applies to your supportive routines and other foundational habits, like eating at set times and regularly relaxing. It's expected that you won't keep up with them perfectly and that you'll have to change your approach till these habits stick better and better.

Similarly, one day you may find a hand-held protector or relaxation technique you've had success with isn't cutting it and that you have to adjust. The next day, it might work again. Reassessing is also about making sure protectors are a fit *that day*.

While many protectors will stay steady, some will be like a rotating cast of characters—and that's OK. Embrace it.

◆

While logging, you may start going through the motions, answering the same way every time. If you get complacent, aim to do more. Really think about the questions rather than assume the trigger or protector is what you think, and that you simply failed—that there's nothing you can do, no way to protect.

Because there is.

When you start to think there isn't is when you're in trouble.

It's just that failing is part of learning.

Each and every time you fail, learn from it; reassess your responsive habits, lifestyle habits, and barriers.

Edit your Protectors List as your knowledge of your BFRB grows.

Do Your Best During Tough Times

Examples of what I call "tough times" include:

- For the duration of some big life event (e.g., a move, a relationship change, a loss)
- During family visits, vacations, and gatherings (e.g., holidays, birthdays, weddings)
- During a significant national or world-wide event
- For the duration of a big project or college exams

During these times, you may have more distress than normal. New triggers may crop up. Urges may be stronger, as you have less bandwidth for even the bare minimum tasks of your day, much less protective, foundational habits, like eating a healthy meal, getting good sleep, journaling, or decompressing, that have you going above and beyond and which keep urges at bay.

Unfortunately, **when we're most tempted to throw these protectors out the window is when we most need them.**

When we're low, we crave comfort food, we don't care as much about our health or goals, we desire a distraction no matter the cost.

Because the toughest time to choose change is when you're low, if you do keep yourself from a destructive habit then, that's a huge gain for your rewiring. (This goes for smoking, drinking, binging, and more, not just BFRBs.)

Sometimes, though, it seems all we can manage is to just hang on, to get by, and that's OK. Do your best during tough times, ride it out, and especially now, have compassion over your BFRB and see protecting as self-care if at all possible.

With practice, you'll come to know yourself better and have a solid enough foundation and arsenal of protectors so that, more and more often, tough times will be no big deal, or they'll at least be manageable.

◆

Fingers are *repeatedly* searching for targets as you keep angling to escape.

You didn't sleep enough.

Because you can't go back in time and sleep more, you can't protect directly from the trigger of being tired. You could nap, but say you have (or want) to work.

Not being able to apply the best or most direct protector is another example of facing "tough times" with your BFRB.

Even if you don't have access to the best protector, though, you *can* address a looming trigger in one way or another. To continue with the example of not having slept enough, you might:

- Coach yourself with counter thoughts.
- Wear gloves.

During tough times, call in heavy-duty barriers, like gloves, covering mirrors, or removing bulbs, that may not be practical for everyday life.

- Move around or step outside to get fresh air and wake you up.
- Drink water, green tea, or coffee (e.g., allow an extra cup of coffee on a day like today).
- Consider doing all of the above.

Layering the protection is always a good idea, not least during tough times.

◆

Other times when things may be tough with your BFRB are related directly to your healing journey, for example when:

- You're going through **trial and error** as you continue to figure out a certain trigger and learn from the failures.
- You're **beginning** or progressing with these steps.

For me, the very beginning of this process was so easy and exciting, I felt like I'd never pick again. But once the high dulled, I was once more worried I'd never be able to stop.

That's because though I was doing better than ever, I was focusing on my skin picking and my triggers—*my "problems"*—more than ever.

This highlighted how often my body wanted to engage in my BFRB, how easily I could become stressed, scattered, or anxious.

All at once, the things I had been escaping were laid bare, **asking to be addressed in a real way**, rather than being pushed away by picking. But thanks to my new awareness and knowledge, I was more capable of doing something.

> *Sometimes things get tougher before they get better.*

Put Your Willpower Here

Earlier I said willpower comes into play later, once you have more advanced tools.

Now is that time.

Willpower and determination alone have *never* been enough. We've already covered that. So if and when this process is hard, do not return to the old pattern of just determining to not pick.

Put your willpower into foundational and responsive habits, as well as barriers. Willpower is meant to *help you protect*, nothing more.

◆

A level of willpower *is* needed to retract your hand, to not lean in, to choose *rewiring* when you're facing down the edge of the cliff. Sure, call willpower in then. It may turn out in your favor, and it's a good move for your healing.

But the willpower needed to protect from a trigger or precursor you notice far on the horizon is much less than the amount needed to *turn around* at the edge of the cliff, and infinitely less than the amount needed to heave yourself up once you've fallen over and have started engaging in your behavior. So **focus your willpower on not being in that situation in the first place**, into staying as far from the edge as possible.

This is the path of least resistance.

◆

Not understanding their BFRB problem, some BFRBers feel like they're not accomplishing anything of their own merit if, for example, they're using barriers (*I'm only doing well because I'm wearing a hat*), or because they have nothing to pick in that moment (perhaps due to improved skin care or diet).

If this is you, be glad for any edge you have over your BFRB!

You pick because your neural pathways toward picking are deeply ingrained, because you have a body-focused repetitive behavior, not because you aren't strong enough to *just not pick*.

In other words, not picking due to a great show of willpower isn't your achievement. Protecting so that you can rewire is.

That's you showing your strength. That's something to really be proud of.

Prioritize Your Healing

If your healing isn't at the top, you might put yourself in a triggering situation to meet a deadline, to please others, or just because you'd rather do something other than care for yourself.

> *Speaking of others, it doesn't matter what anyone thinks about the choices you make for your BFRB healing, be it in regard to protective foundational habits or barriers. The things you have to do for yourself are between you and you.*

Perhaps your BFRB *won't* be at the very top every day—maybe an important deadline must be met, maybe your sobriety from drugs or alcohol is your number one. But on most days, place your healing near the very top of your priorities, if not in the number one spot.

Keep Protecting

If you find yourself ignoring your protectors, look at *why* that is. Why is this time an exception to protecting?

Maybe you feel you can have the bathroom light on *this* time. You might remember when you were able to defy a protector and *not* pick (though it was probably because you didn't have many triggers that day). For example, you went into the bathroom, flicked on the light, checked yourself out, and walked away. You may use that as a reason to ignore protectors at whim, forgetting all the many more times bypassing a protector failed you. For example, you went into the bathroom, flicked on the light, got sucked into the mirror, and picked badly.

For a while, I would consciously ignore my protectors and pick a little. Because I was doing so *well*, I felt like it was OK, that I was in control. But I wasn't. Not anymore. With that mentality, I had steered back into the weeds of the dermatillo-*mania* mind.

As one skin picker said, that 1% of times it went OK is all we remember. We selectively conclude something that catapults us into picking, while putting aside everything we've learned that goes against it.

Only *after* the consequences are staring us down do we remember the 99% of the time we regretted picking.

So keep in place all those wonderful protectors you've brainstormed.

No matter what.

Be devoted. Be diligent. Be strict.

Stay in the mindset of healing.

You'll soon be able to compare the wonderful progress you make when you're on your toes with protectors versus when you're lenient.

You'll see how wonderful you look and feel, and you'll *want* to practice your protectors.

◆

Can't stop, or progress came but now you're backsliding?

Ask yourself:

Have you truly worked on cementing a healthy foundation in the first place? Your dermatillomania won't heal itself. You must do the work, even if it's by putting down tiny foundational blocks.

Did you start and then give up on your routines, on your basics, on more helpful patterns of thinking? If yes, it's understandable, since old wiring has momentum on any new pathways, but little by little, take these habits back up.

◆

You have a leg up on others, because now that you know these concepts, increased picking will send you a clear wake-up and remind you to practice protectors.

So, stay with protectors. You're on the right track. You've arrived. It's just a matter of practicing till you get it right.

Add New Items to Your Log

Let's add new items to your log. Soon I'll explain how these will take your healing even further as you round out the guide.

Please, get out your notebook, or open your note app. I'll wait.

Session Questions

Add these new items to your session questions:

- Do I know my trigger(s)? (Shorthand can be *Triggers?*)
- What can I do next time? (*Do next time?*)
- How can I protect now? (*Protect now?*)
- Any new triggers or protectors to list? (*List anything?*)

Urge Questions

Because you can log when you're triggered too, not only when it's become an *outright* desire to pick or pull (an urge), change this heading to **Urge/Trigger**. Then add the same questions from above to this set of questions too.

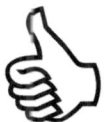

Here's a breakdown of how these help:

Do I Know My Trigger(s)?

Answering these new questions will get you out of autopilot and help you identify further triggers, even if you've already discovered some while answering the earlier questions.

> *At different times, certain log questions, like this one, will be more and less useful.*

What Can I Do Next Time?

Imagine yourself in the same situation—going to the start of the chain of events, what would you have done differently to prevent this session, triggering situation, or urge?

This question is to brainstorm *new* protectors and practice existing ones, as it helps you remember and ingrain them.

It can also get you to tweak and improve what you've been doing.

How Can I Protect Now?

It might seem pointless to protect *after* picking, but suppose that relaxing is how you decide you can protect; this will reduce the chance of further picking, be it for that day (*since, even after a session, the desire to escape may persist*) or the next (*since this relaxation will trickle into the following day*).

Protecting even after a session is smart!

And when logging an urge, this question is extra useful, since it can *prevent* a session.

Any New Triggers or Protectors to List?

You don't have to write anything here, though you can. This is to remind you to open up your Triggers and/or Protectors Lists if you *have* discovered something new to list.

Your Current Log

At this point, your log will look something like this:

DATE?

TIME? | HOW LONG?

AREAS?

DOING BEFORE?

FELT BEFORE?

FELT DURING?

FELT AFTER?

TRIGGER(S)?

DO NEXT TIME?

PROTECT NOW?

LIST ANYTHING?

    URGE/TRIGGER

DATE?

TIME?

DOING WHAT?

FEELING WHAT?

TRIGGER(S)?

DO NEXT TIME?

PROTECT NOW?

LIST ANYTHING?

A Final Word on Step 4

Knowing your BFRB is on the horizon is such a huge step that it might feel like your work is done, but part of practicing protectors is taking the next step:

Which is to *do something*. To act. To actually protect.

Don't go through your day with a nagging urge as your passenger. Don't ignore, deny, suppress, or resist a trigger or urge. This is the old way, and remember, it doesn't work.

The new way is to figure out what you need to do for yourself, and **then to do it.**

◆

Your relationship with your BFRB when you've only begun these steps will be much different compared to when you've been following them for a while.

Once your awareness becomes keen, your Triggers List becomes vast, and your protectors are practiced, *that's* when the healing you see will excite you.

You won't visit the other steps as much once your footing with your healing gets firmer. Step 4, Practice Protectors, is where you'll live.

Post Steps

Track Your Improvement
How Long Does This Take?
What Healing Means
Relapse
When to Stop Following These Steps
More Logging and Listing Options

Track Your Improvement

While tracking isn't necessary for healing, it can help. Because BFRBers can be perfectionists and relapse can have us feeling like we've made no progress at all, tracking can show you how far you've truly come, which can encourage you forward.

Also, over time, you'll see trends relating to work, school, family, and more and how much or how little you picked, offering clues as to which areas of your life require changes or added protection.

In the beginning, I focused on healing without thinking about whether I was doing better or worse than I thought, hoped, or expected. However, for some, a running tally from the start *may* be helpful. Maybe you have a competitive spirit and want to actively strive to keep your number as low as possible.

If you start tracking now and your numbers begin to distress you, though, put them on the back burner. Over time, your hair, nails, lips—your mood and more—will show you progress. When they do, try tracking again.

If you're unsure, start tracking your improvement now and then pause it or keep it up, depending on whether it's helpful or not.

How to Track

To see your progress, you'll compare one month to the next, so at the *first* of the following month:

- Go through your log and add up the numbers under **How Long?**

*Entries labeled **Urge/Trigger** will not go toward this tracking.*

This will show you approximately for how long you engaged in your behavior for that month. Next month, do the same thing.

◆

Though every tracking method has its limitations, time is a better metric than counting the number of sessions or the days in which you pick. If you see you still pick daily, or that you do it several times a day, that can be discouraging, but this doesn't take into account that *not all sessions are equal*: that is, even if you still pick frequently, you may be picking for radically less time.

Gauge Improvement Over Time

So that you can see the big picture, you'll record the amount you pick month over month.

I recommend either a list and/or a graph for this record. Either way, create this space now, so you have it ready for when you need it.

List

With a list, you'll end up with something that looks like:

Tracking Improvement
- April 2024 – # hrs. # min.
- May 2024 – # hrs. # min.
- June 2024 – # hrs. # min.

 # will be replaced with actual figures.

To create a list:

- Create a new **note app note**, and update it every month.
- Clip a fresh sheet into your **physical notebook**, and update it every month.

Graph

You can also create a line graph that looks something like:

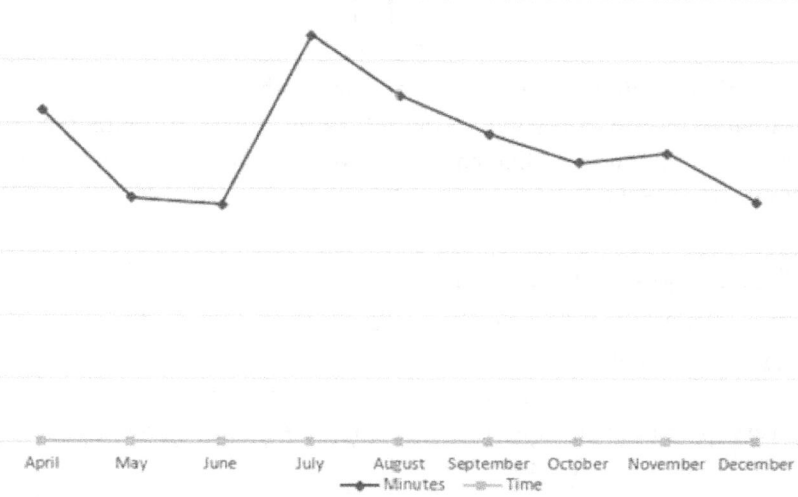

Your graph will show actual figures.

To create a graph:

- Use **Excel on a computer**. (This is what I recommend.)

    Excel is easy enough to figure out if you work with computers here and there.

- Download a **graph app** for your phone.

    If you find these difficult, try using Excel on a computer.

- Create a graph with **pencil and paper**, whether you use a ruler and plain paper or graph paper.

Staple or paper-clip this graph into your BFRB notebook; if you use a note app, keep this graph somewhere handy.

It's unlikely you started logging on the first of the month, so add up this initial month to give you a sense of how much you currently pick or pull, but leave it out when comparing your progress from one month to the next in the future.

Goals and No-Pick Challenges

Once you have some data, you can use it to create specific, attainable goals, if you'd like.

For example, at some point in my own healing, I realized I'd pick every three days. It could be for just a minute—but I'd pick. It seemed I never made it past three.

So I created a four-day challenge (notice I made the goal attainable—I didn't do, say, a month-long challenge). More strides in healing happened this way.

This is one idea you may like.

Another is to aim to reduce the time you pick next month compared to this month. But remember to be specific and to make it attainable. For example, how much would you like to reduce it by? Twenty or thirty minutes? An hour? What one thing can you do to help this happen?

Make sure you have a solid understanding of the steps before goal-setting. Otherwise, you may begin to use sheer force of will to keep you from picking, and as covered, that won't work.

How Long Does This Take?

I wouldn't want to give you a time frame that makes you think (consciously or subconsciously) something like: *It hasn't been long enough. I must be about to mess up, because I'm not supposed to be healed yet.*

Or, *It's taking longer than it was supposed to. Maybe I'll never get to the point I want. Maybe I'm more messed up than others.*

Not at all.

Think about how long you've been picking, pulling, or biting. It won't take nearly that long to see significant healing, but it may put a time frame into perspective.

So, how long will it take for you to see significant healing? *Some time* is all I can say. With these steps and any other process, picking tends to *lessen over time*, dropping sharply at first, and then going through peaks and valleys depending on what your life looks like (e.g., tough times versus low-stress times) **and how well you're following these steps.**

Stretched out over a period, it might look like this, with bad months followed by better ones and excellent months followed by poor ones, till things eventually even out:

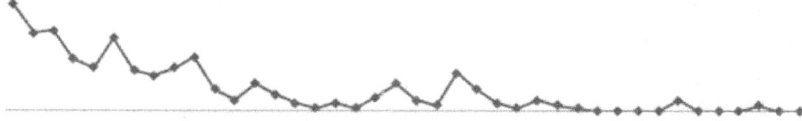

Healing is not linear. Indeed, as with most issues in life, it's more of a meandering, self-growth type of deal.

And even then, the process may never be over *fully*. A few examples of why that is:

- Even once you've got a handle on your BFRB, you may discover a new trigger—one that didn't even exist before, or which never came up before, for which you must now establish protectors.
- You may experience a hormonal shift or a life-altering event that has you regaining your footing.

However, having a BFRB is not just about the picking or pulling itself. Desperation and helplessness are a huge part of it. These steps will give you something even more satisfying than nicer skin, hair, or nails (though you'll get that too). You'll get control—power. And that comes much sooner.

What Healing Means

Those of us on the other side of the BFRB problem may use words like "stop" and "heal" to communicate efficiently with those who aren't here yet because these are the words you understand—possibly the only words you're willing to hear. If we don't use those words, you might not listen: "No, no, I want to *stop*. How do I do *that*?"

But a word like "manage" is appropriate for most.

When I say I'm healed I mean that I'm managing my skin picking extremely well, that it's not a problem for me anymore. Or if it ever is, it's a much smaller one than it ever was. It's one I have control over.

Some *can* stop unwanted behaviors completely and suddenly through an epiphany or perspective-rocking event or piece of knowledge, but many BFRBers who consider themselves recovered, including me, sometimes still pick, pull, or chew, if here and there.

I'm still practicing and fine-tuning protectors, and I go through my own tough times in life.

But don't get me wrong.

My dermatillomania today and my dermatillomania before are completely different. I sometimes forget a failure used to be having a red, raw face, back, legs, chest. *Hours* wasted, rather than minutes. The disorder that assailed me for seventeen years has *radically* improved, and it's still getting better.

The incredible reduction I've had in my BFRB is one of my greatest personal achievements. At times, I'm still amazed, because of how impossible it once felt.

So, is stopping 100% possible?

It's what I'm aiming for.

I think it's possible due to how far I've gotten, and I'd like to add that this aim is also important to my healing. The moment I aim any lower than zero picking, my *mania* mind takes over, and my picking gets out of hand. But this isn't the same for everyone. I know of those who are satisfied with a high degree of healing, and those who've already stopped completely.

◆

I don't want the idea of not stopping 100%, right away or forevermore, to scare you from these steps or any other process. I promise walking onto the path of healing is worth it. I've never spoken to a recovered BFRBer who doesn't agree.

Relapse

Once you've gone a day, week, month, or more without significant picking or pulling, when—if—you do pick or pull badly, it may feel like a new kind of failure and possibly be more distressing than when you used to give in *before* these steps.

At least that's how it was for me.

But I never found it useful to decide I was "starting over." That wiped out the progress I *had* made. It gave me anxiety that made me crave to pick more. I'd get lazy with my protectors, feeling there was no point, because I'd never reach perfection. (Now I know that's not what healing means anyway.) It felt more encouraging to say that I was still on the path of healing. This made me remember protectors, regain the feeling of being healed. I could put aside that old feeling, which came up during the relapse, of being stuck.

I could tune in to my new story again.

You may think about this differently. Some like to think of themselves as being allowed to start over whenever, to start over hundreds of times if necessary, to have a clean slate at whim.

Regardless of how you see it, your progress is yours forever.

◆

The pain over your BFRB has served its purpose: to push you to change. Similarly, the heavy feeling after slips and relapses is good for getting you to recommit to protectors, and to yourself. When you fall back, let those negative emotions propel you that many steps *and more* forward.

That's all these emotions are for.

Personally, I'm at my most committed when I have just slipped or relapsed. If this is you too, why not harness this time for some concentrated rewiring, for some diligent practice of protectors?

As covered in Step 4, through every slip or relapse, strive to learn something to use in your healing. **This is how you make sure a relapse doesn't go to waste.**

If you do pick or pull, try not to feed the old energy and story. Things are different now. You know what you need to do now.

Love yourself, be kind to yourself, and be on your side, even in those moments of relapse.

When to Stop Following These Steps

Your healing is contained in three spots: your log and two lists. I recommend you keep it there.

Personally, I haven't been healed from my BFRB for nearly as long as I struggled with it (almost two decades), so I will keep logging for the foreseeable future. To this day, I still discover triggers, protectors, and insights while doing so.

I might need to keep my barriers in place for quite a long time, and it's possible that I'll always have to avoid certain triggering actions, such as leaning too close to the mirror or running my hands over bumps. That makes sense to me. And of course, many protective responsive and foundational habits are just part of a happy life, BFRB or not.

That said, some skin pickers stop logging and listing when they feel firmly recovered.

If you do this, and you start slipping back, **return to this process**. Pick up logging and listing where you left off. Try protectors that you weren't drawn to before. Re-read the entire guide, or parts of it, to remind yourself of the concepts or to soak them in more deeply.

Concepts that seem obvious as you read about them may fall to the back of your mind by the time you're living your daily life. Even though I tried to make this simple—there's a lot to it.

However, this guide will always be here for you.

I welcome you to use the BFRB Guide as a reference text, revisiting it as needed, possibly often.

More Logging and Listing Options

The purpose of the log is to *identify triggers and perfect protectors*. Now that you know this, feel free to find ways to make that process work better for you. Here are some ideas:

- Log in your regular journal—so, by the time the journal is filled, it'll have regular entries peppered with BFRB entries. Use some marking, color, or symbol that calls it out as a BFRB entry, in case you ever want to review your entries.

    Re-reading your log entries can offer even more insight into your BFRB and show you how far you've progressed. You don't have to, but you might like to.

- Keep your triggers and protectors in **one** list, rather than two, e.g., have only one note for this in your note app.
- Split your lists further, e.g., create a note for separate categories.
- Keep your log and/or lists in a binder with loose-leaf paper.

> Above all, it's important you have some log and list method set up and that it's workable enough to support your healing, even if it's not perfect.

If in doubt, log and list as instructed. As you learn more about your personal healing process, change up your system, if you'd like.

A Final Word on the Guide

Sometimes, we're not ready to heal or change. Whether we realize it or not, a diagnosis or behavior—some story—can become such a part of how we see ourselves or how we present ourselves to others that we might not want to let it go.

Or we want an instant cure. Or we expect someone, maybe a

therapist, coach, or loved one, to save us, make it go away, or fix it for us (not yet understanding that the change must ultimately come from us).

But often, it's not that BFRBers aren't ready or willing to stop, they just don't know how.

Now you do.

◆

My hope is that you will do so much more than just enjoy your improved skin, hair, or nails.

Take the confidence that comes with stopping your skin picking disorder, your trichotillomania, or whatever your BFRB happens to be and use it to level up, to be your best self, to seek more connection, fulfillment, financial security—whatever you want.

And, if you'd like, after you change your world for the better, take on the whole world.

End

Endnotes (Sources by Section)
Selected Bibliography
Resources
Acknowledgments
About the Author
Contact
More BFRB Guide
Review & Recommend

Endnotes

Sources by Section

I believe in giving credit where credit is due. I thank these sources for making their wisdom accessible. (Also see Selected Bibliography.)

Pre-Steps

1. S. H. Young, "The Complete Guide to Self-Control," Sep 2019, accessed Sep 2019.
2. M. Rodrigues, "Health Check: Is It Bad to Pop Your Pimples?" The Conversation, Mar 20, 2016, accessed Jan 26, 2021.
Also: A. Diaz and J. Zeichner, "The Reason Why You Keep Getting Pimples in the Same Place," The Klog, Dec 16, 2020, accessed Jan 25, 2021.
3. Diaz and Zeichner, "The Reason Why You Keep Getting Pimples in the Same Place."
4. Diaz and Zeichner, "The Reason Why You Keep Getting Pimples in the Same Place."
5. D. Kern, "What Causes a Pimple to Scar?" Acne.org, Feb 18, 2021, accessed Feb 20, 2021.
6. C. Novak, "Everything You Always Wanted to Know About Hair . . . But Were Afraid to Ask," Community Resource Library, The TLC Foundation for BFRBs, accessed Jan 26, 2021.
7. D. Kern, "How Long Does It Take for a Pimple to Form?" Acne.org, updated Feb 18, 2021, accessed Feb 20, 2021.
8. A. Mattu and A. Curcio, "Self-Compassion and Acceptance: The Building Blocks of Change with Dr. Ali Mattu," The TLC Foundation for BFRBs, webinar, attended Jun 25, 2020, recording can be accessed on YouTube, time stamp 1:10.

9. American Psychiatric Association, *Diagnostic and Statistical Manual of Mental Disorders: Fifth Edition* (Arlington, VA: American Psychiatric Association Publishing, 2013), 235–237.
10. A. Mattu and A. Curcio, "Self-Compassion and Acceptance: The Building Blocks of Change with Dr. Ali Mattu," The TLC Foundation for BFRBs, webinar, attended Jun 25, 2020, recording can be accessed on YouTube, time stamp 1:12.

The Steps

1. K. Martinko, "'Niksen' Is the Delightful Dutch Concept of Doing Nothing," Treehugger, Oct 11, 2018, accessed Aug 27, 2020.
2. "The Science of Gratitude," Tremendousness, accessed Oct 24, 2020.
3. A. Park, "This Is the Fastest Way to Calm Down," *Time* magazine, Mar 30, 2017, accessed Oct 14, 2020.
Also: M. Zetlin, "Neuroscience Just Explained Why This Simple Technique for Calm and Mental Focus Works So Well," Inc.com, Nov 12, 2018, accessed Oct 18, 2020.
4. S. Baxter, "How to Relieve Stress and Anxiety Fast (Somatic Practice)," video, Oct 12, 2020, accessed Jan 5, 2021.
5. S. Jacoby and E. Newsom, "This Is How Often You Should Actually Exfoliate Your Face," SELF, Feb 22, 2019, accessed Jan 4, 2021.
6. K. Hanson, "How Do the Chemicals in Sunscreen Protect Our Skin from Damage?" The Conversation, May 25, 2017, accessed Mar 7, 2021.
7. Cancer Council Australia, "10 Myths About Sun Protection," accessed Feb 17, 2021.
8. R. Mawer, "17 Proven Tips to Sleep Better at Night," Healthline, Feb 28, 2020, accessed Jan 20, 2021.
9. S. Okimi, C. Heath, and H. Mitchell, "Grow Edges Back Fast | Real Dermatologists Tell All," video, Feb 4, 2021, accessed Feb 5, 2021.
10. M. Guido, "Common Causes of Dry Hair and Scalp + Solutions," video, Feb 25, 2020, accessed Feb 4, 2021, time stamp 12:28.
11. Guido, "Common Causes of Dry Hair and Scalp + Solutions," time stamp 1:15.

12. "7 Dermatologists' Tips for Healing Dry, Chapped Lips," American Academy of Dermatology Association, accessed Feb 4, 2021.
13. J. E. Grant, S. R. Chamberlain, S. A. Redden, et al, "N-Acetylcysteine in the Treatment of Excoriation Disorder: A Randomized Clinical Trial," *JAMA Psychiatry*, 2016;73(5), 490–496.

    Also: J. E. Grant, B. L. Odlaug, S. W. Kim, "N-Acetylcysteine, a Glutamate Modulator, in the Treatment of Trichotillomania: A Double-Blind, Placebo-Controlled Study," *Archives of General Psychiatry*, Jul 2009, 66(7), 756–763.
14. R. Richter, "Antioxidants Help Treat Skin-Picking Disorder in Mice," Stanford Medicine News Center, Jul 13, 2015, accessed Jan 12, 2021.
15. İ. Akaltun, "Trichotillomania Triggered by Vitamin D Deficiency and Resolving Dramatically with Vitamin D Therapy," *Clinical Neuropharmacology*, Jan/Feb 2019, 42(1), 20–21.
16. J. W. Skelley, C. M. Deas, Z. Curren, and J. Ennis, "Use of Cannabidiol in Anxiety and Anxiety-Related Disorders," Journal of the American Pharmacists Association: JAPhA, Nov 19, 2019, 253–61.
17. SciLit (Scientific Literacy) Journal Club, The TLC Foundation for BFRBs, webinar/meeting, attended Jan 18, 2021, recording can be accessed on YouTube, time stamp 0:50.

    Also: "BFRB Precision Medicine Update," The TLC Foundation for BFRBs (Scientific Advisory Board), webinar, attended Dec 8, 2020, recording can be accessed on YouTube.
18. K. Shkodzik, "Hormonal Imbalance in Women: 9 Signs to Look For," Jan 19, 2021, accessed Feb 5, 2021.
19. "What Multitasking Does to Your Brain," BBC Ideas, video, Apr 28, 2020, accessed Feb 5, 2021.
20. R. Ryback, "The Science of Accomplishing Your Goals," Psychology Today, Oct 3, 2016, accessed Mar 8, 2021.
21. J. Bell, "How to Develop Confidence When You Feel Worthless, According to Science," Big Think, Mar 6, 2020, accessed Oct 20, 2020.
22. A. Brenner, "The Inner Language of the Subconscious," Psychology Today, Jan 29, 2013, accessed Jan 20, 2021.
23. E. Suni and E. Callender, "What Happens When You Sleep?" SleepFoundation.org, Oct 30, 2020, accessed Mar 9, 2021.

Also: E. Suni and A. Dimitriu, "Mental Health and Sleep," SleepFoundation.org, Sep 18, 2020, accessed Mar 9, 2021.
24. "Nutrition and Wound Healing," Nutrition Education Materials Online, Apr 2017, accessed Feb 17, 2021.
25. E. L. Guo and R. Katta. "Diet and Hair Loss: Effects of Nutrient Deficiency and Supplement Use," *Dermatology Practical & Conceptual*, 2017, 7(1), 1–10.
26. M. Oaklander and H. Jones, "7 Surprising Benefits of Exercise," *Time* magazine, Sep 1, 2016, accessed Feb 20, 2021.
27. E. Suni and A. Singh, "How Much Sleep Do We Really Need?" SleepFoundation.org, Jul 31, 2020, accessed Feb 17, 2021.
28. C. P. Landrigan, "Assess Your Sleep Needs," Division of Sleep Medicine at Harvard Medical School, Dec 15, 2008, accessed Feb 17, 2021.
29. Suni and Singh, "How Much Sleep Do We Really Need?"
30. Institute of Medicine (US) Committee on Sleep Medicine and Research, H. R. Colten and B. M. Altevogt, editors, *Sleep Disorders and Sleep Deprivation: An Unmet Public Health Problem* (Washington, DC: National Academies Press, US, 2006), 63.
31. L. J. Epstein, "Adopt Good Sleep Habits," Division of Sleep Medicine at Harvard Medical School, Dec 12, 2008, accessed Feb 17, 2021.
32. S. Egan, "Making the Case for Eating Fruit," *New York Times Magazine*, Jul 31, 2013, accessed Nov 19, 2020.
33. J. Fuhrman, *Eat to Live* (New York: Little, Brown & Company, 2011), 92.
34. Fuhrman, 11.
35. R. Link, "8 Health Benefits of Fasting, Backed by Science," Healthline, Jul 30, 2018, accessed Mar 9, 2021.
36. T. Raftl, "The Love Vitamin's Guide to Eating Dairy When You've Got Acne," The Love Vitamin blog, accessed Sep 7, 2020.
37. M. Greger, "If Fructose Is Bad, What About Fruit?" video, Dec 3, 2014, accessed Oct 28, 2020, time stamp 3:09.
38. M. Greger, "How to Prevent Blood Sugar and Triglyceride Spikes after Meals," video, Apr 19, 2017, accessed Mar 9, 2021, time stamp 2:16.

39. R. Jordan, "Stanford Researchers Find Mental Health Prescription: Nature," Stanford News, Jun 30, 2015, accessed Mar 8, 2021.
40. R. Halliwell, "Why Dancing Feels So Good," The Telegraph, Apr 29, 2016, accessed Feb 8, 2021.
41. R. Poldrack, "Multitasking: The Brain Seeks Novelty," HuffPost blog, Nov 17, 2011, accessed Mar 7, 2021.

Selected Bibliography

Rather than citing one piece of information from the following sources, I wove their wisdom throughout.

Garner, C. and Curcio, A. "4 Steps to Melt Your Urges on the Spot." The TLC Foundation for BFRBs. Webinar series, attended Apr–May 2020. A full list of the webinars and recordings can be found on the TLC site.

Miletíc, V. "Exploring Hair Pulling Trances." TrichStop Online Therapy. Webinar, attended on Oct 21, 2020. Recording can be accessed on YouTube.

Miletíc, V. "Habit Reversal Training for Hair Pulling." TrichStop Online Therapy. Webinar, attended on Nov 13, 2020. Recording can be accessed on YouTube.

Miletíc, V. "Making and Breaking Habits." TrichStop Online Therapy. Webinar, attended on Sep 18, 2020. Recording can be accessed on YouTube.

Resources

I do not support, nor am I aware of, every statement, view, or opinion by the following organizations and persons, but I believe you'll find use in at least some, if not much, of their material.

BFRB Support

- The TLC Foundation | Authoritative BFRB information and news on the latest research. Support groups and webinars available.
- Picking Me Foundation | A donor-supported non-profit for skin picking. Support groups and fun activities available.
- Obsessive Skin Pickers Anonymous (OSPA) | Those who enjoy 12-step programs may benefit from connecting with other BFRBers through OSPA.

OCD & Anxiety

- OCD Center of LA | BFRB info is available, but their OCD and anxiety support in particular is excellent.

BFRB Supplements & Avoiding Toxicity

- Article: "N-acetylcysteine for Trichotillomania, Skin Picking, and Nail Biting"
- Earth Working Group (EWG) | An independent non-profit providing trustworthy info on living healthier.

Blemishes & Skin Care

- Dr. Dray on YouTube
- Team Acne on YouTube
- TheLoveVitamin.com
- Expert Advice articles by Paula's Choice

Productivity & Time Management

- Scott H. Young's site
- How to ADHD on YouTube
- muchelleb on YouTube

Habits

- *Atomic Habits* by James Clear
- *The Power of Habit* by Charles Duhigg

Acknowledgments

A loving thank-you to Teresa and Jeffery Gerade for their endless support; to Matthew Mitchell for providing wonderful feedback and support; to my family, especially my mom, Mercedes Bloise De Meira; and, not least, to that part of me that never lets me give up.

About the Author

Originally from the tropical island of Dominican Republic, Lauren Inés Ruiz Bloise is a writer, editor, designer, Spanish–English medical interpreter, and recovered skin picker. She currently lives in New Hampshire in the USA.

Contact

If you have questions, comments, or concerns, email me at **contact@healyourBFRB.com**. Don't worry about how many emails I may be getting—I want your message in my inbox.

More BFRB Guide

Visit the online home of the BFRB Guide at **healyourBFRB.com**.

Join the email list, follow on social media, and favorite on Etsy to be alerted of upcoming products and projects.

I welcome you to inquire about BFRB coaching, which I offer periodically throughout the year.

Review & Recommend

If this guide helped you, please **leave a review** wherever you purchased it and **recommend** it to those you think it may help. Thank you!

www.ingramcontent.com/pod-product-compliance
Lightning Source LLC
LaVergne TN
LVHW051114080426
835510LV00018B/2026